MRCP 2
Success in PACES

Philip Kelly
Specialist Registrar in Endocrinology,
St Bartholomew's Hospital
and The Royal London Hospital

Thomas Powles
Specialist Registrar in Medical Oncology,
St Bartholomew's Hospital and
the Royal London Hospital

and

Paul Jenkins
Reader in Endocrinology and Consultant Physician,
St Bartholomew's Hospital and
The Royal London Hospital

PASTEST
Dedicated to your success

© 2003 PasTest Ltd
Egerton Court
Parkgate Estate
Knutsford
Cheshire WA16 8DX

Telephone: 01565 752000

First edition 2003

ISBN: 1 901198 685

A catalogue record for this book is available from the British Library.

The information contained within this book was obtained by the authors from reliable sources. However, while every effort has been made to ensure its accuracy, no responsibility for loss, damage or injury occasioned to any person acting or refraining from action as a result of information contained herein can be accepted by the publisher or the authors.

PasTest Revision Books and Intensive Courses
PasTest has been established in the field of postgraduate medical education since 1972, providing revision books and intensive study courses for doctors preparing for their professional examinations. Books and courses are available for the following specialties:

MRCP Part 1 and Part 2, MRCPCH Part 1 and Part 2, MRCS, MRCOG, DRCOG, MRCGP, MRCPsych, DCH, FRCA and PLAB

For further details contact:

PasTest, Freepost, Knutsford, Cheshire WA16 7BR
Tel: 01565 752 000   Fax: 01565 650 264
Email: enquiries@pastest.co.uk   Web site: www. pastest.co.uk

Typeset by Saxon Graphics Ltd, Derby
Printed and bound in Great Britain by Page Bros (Norwich) Ltd

Contents

The authors dedicate this book to their teachers, colleagues and families.

Philip Kelly
Thomas Powles
Paul Jenkins

Acknowledgements

The authors gratefully acknowledge the assistance of the following colleagues:
Mike Arden Jones, James Bower, Claire Hemmaway, Sarah Howling, Mark Nelson, Fergus Robertson and Deborah Ruddy for their invaluable help.

Introduction

GENERAL POINTS

The clinical part of the MRCP (UK) Part 2 PACES – Practical Assessment of Clinical Examination Skills – is a demanding and difficult examination, but overall a fair one. It must first of all be emphasised that the examiners are not looking for the next Professor of Medicine, but rather a safe and competent doctor, who is suitable for higher specialist training. Examiners say time and time again that their criteria for passing an examinee are based on whether they would entrust the care of one of their relatives to the candidate. Alternatively, would they be able to have a sensible and practical conversation if the candidate, as their specialist registrar, rang in the early hours of the morning regarding a patient? However, as with the previous parts of the examination, a pass is the result of successful examination technique together with clinical skills and knowledge. Communicating to the examiners that you are safe, competent and knowledgeable is a vital component of the examination. Careful preparation is therefore essential as you are being tested on both examination technique and presentation skills. All too often candidates fail themselves through the lack of self-belief that they are able to pass the exam and adopting the 'rabbit caught in the headlights' stance. It is vital to remember the key words of 'confidence' and 'competence'.

GENERAL APPROACH

Remember that the examiners are trying to find out what you know and are not trying to catch you out. Their brief is to determine whether you are suitable for specialist training.

Approach the examiners in a friendly and confident manner, although, obviously, overfamiliarity or arrogance are a sure way to antagonise. When discussing the patient do so in an interested manner, as you would when talking to your consultant or another senior colleague and not as a first-year medical student talking to the Professor. Dress smartly and conservatively. Do not smell of cigarettes, aftershave or alcohol. Eye contact is an important part of communication and should be appropriately maintained with the examiners. Far too many candidates enter the 'victim mode', with arms folded, eyes downcast, almost expecting to fail. Do not do this. Keep your hands by your sides or behind your back, where fidgeting or finger twisting will not be noticed. Remember, people all too often fail themselves in this exam, despite being a good clinician in their normal hospital. The exam is both easy to pass and easy to fail.

Treat the patients with respect and consideration at all times. Remember, they have given their time freely. There is no easier way of failing than inadvertently hurting a patient during clumsy examination of a limb or abdominal system. Always ask the patient if they have any pain or tenderness before you put 'hands on'.

Finally, prepare for the exam carefully. If you have failed the exam previously make sure you know the reason why. Identify those areas in which you are weak and make sure that you see as many cases as you can, preferably in exam conditions.

ABOUT THE EXAMINATION

Exam content

The PACES examination consists of five stations, each of 20 minutes' duration, and with 5 minutes rest/preparation between stations.

- Station 1 – Respiratory and abdominal examination (10 minutes each)
- Station 2 – History-taking examination (20 minutes)
- Station 3 – Cardiovascular and neurological examination (10 minutes each)
- Station 4 – Communication skills and ethics' examination (20 minutes)
- Station 5 – Skin, locomotor, eye and endocrine examination (5 minutes each)

Stations 1 and 3

Candidates will respond to written instructions. After 5 minutes of examination, candidates will be asked to complete the clinical examination to allow for discussion about the case, focusing on investigation and management issues.

Stations 2 and 4

Candidates are given 5 minutes before the station begins in which to review the written scenario and to prepare themselves. They are encouraged to make preparatory notes during this period, but this is not assessed.

The consultation with the patient or subject lasts 14 minutes. This is followed by 1 minute for the candidate to collect their thoughts and then 5 minutes of discussion with the examiners.

Station 5

Candidates will respond to written instructions. Each station lasts for 5 minutes, and interaction with the examiners takes place on a more *ad hoc* basis than in Stations 1 and 3.

Marking

Each candidate will receive 14 structured marking sheets prior to the start of the examination. One sheet is given to each examiner at Stations 2, 4 and 5 and two sheets are given to each examiner at Stations 1 and 3. Examiners record their marks, independently of each other, and place them into a box at the end of the station. There are four possible marks:
- Clear fail = 1 mark
- Fail = 2 marks
- Pass = 3 marks
- Clear pass = 4 marks.

A total of 56 marks is possible. The pass mark is usually set at 42 marks, allowing a pass rate of 45–50%. Any candidate receiving three 'clear fails' automatically fails the examination.

Examination of systems (Stations 1, 3 and 5)

Many candidates find this to be the most difficult and stressful part of the examination. However, with adequate preparation and practice, this should not be the case. Remember that the majority of cases will be patients with chronic stable disease, often encountered in a hospital setting. There are eight clinical examination stations. Be sure that for each system you have your own well-rehearsed method of examination. This is vital, so that if the examiner says, 'Examine the cardiovascular system', or 'Examine the hands' you do not have to think about what to do. The detail of your examination routine should be absolutely auto-matic and look slick and well practised, so that you can concentrate on whether the signs are abnormal or normal. Although there is no completely 'right' examination technique, there are accepted standard methods that one should learn and broadly adhere to.

The majority of patients that one will encounter will have common pathology, e.g. valvular heart disease, diabetic retinopathy, bronchiectasis, arthritides, etc., rather than obscure rarities of tertiary referral centres. It is a common misconception of candidates that esoteric cases are over-represented – imagine you are the registrar calling patients up, and who you might find available with good, stable signs and who is well.

Do your thinking while you are examining the patient; otherwise, when you lift your head from listening to the patient's heart/looking at a fundus and the examiner says, 'Diagnosis?' you will be in difficulty. If you know the diagnosis, it is preferable to continue your presentation by stating it, followed by the relevant supporting clinical findings, e.g. 'This patient has mitral stenosis. The relevant findings are a mitral valvotomy scar; she is in atrial fibrillation with a tapping apex and has a low-pitched mid-diastolic rumbling murmur…'. If you do not know what the diagnosis is, then describe what you see, e.g. 'A rash with plaques involving the trunk and extensor aspects of the elbows' and then give your diagnosis of 'Consistent with psoriasis'. Take charge of the situation and try not to be pressurised. Once you have decided on your findings, stick with them. The examiners may ask you if you are sure: indecision and changing your mind can all too easily lead to floundering and digging yourself a hole, with possibly dire consequences. However, if there is uncertainty, state it, and proceed to say how you would resolve the uncertainty. Present the examiners and thus the patient with a solution, not a problem, and they will be happy.

Concentrate on the current station and the task in hand rather than on perceived mistakes made in previous stations. Although coming up with the right answer is obviously important, the majority of the marks are awarded for overall technique, approach, ability to discuss your findings and clinical judgement, as well as being able to solve clinical problems.

The only way to be confident about the systems examinations is practice, practice and more practice. You should enter the systems examinations as a finely honed diagnostic machine.

History-taking (Station 2)

The history-taking skills' station aims to assess the ability of the candidate to gather data from the patient, to assimilate that data in a structured manner and then to discuss the case in a coherent manner with the examiners. Although the majority of candidates may regard this station as perhaps the easiest, in the exam situation many find this is not the case. A common reason for failure is inadequate preparation and approach, leading to missing out whole sections of a medical history, e.g. drugs, family or social history. The examiners place great emphasis on a careful and thorough social/occupational history. Imagine yourself as the patient and how the illness would affect all the daily activities that you might take for granted, e.g. how does a dialysis patient cope with changing the peritoneal bags, or a rheumatoid arthritic patient cope with dressing and eating, etc.?

Try and cultivate a friendly rapport with your patient and remember that at the end of the history, one should ask, 'Is there anything else that you think I ought to know, or we have not covered?' Often the patient may mention an aspect of the case that is of particular importance which you have overlooked.

You must use the 1 minute after the consultation to collect your thoughts and organise the history in a logical and thoughtful manner. This is not the final MB and the examiners will become irritated by a sloppy presentation with irrelevant negative findings. 'Ums' and 'Uhs' and long pauses do not convey the best image and can be to your detriment. Think and speak clearly, be certain in both your uncertainty and certainty. You should be prepared to discuss the case in relation to the normal presentation of the condition, and to discuss subsequent investigations and treatment. The examiners will expect a considered and mature approach to the case, using a problem-oriented method.

In all aspects of the exam do not start your discussion with the esoteric and obscure, in the belief that you will impress the examiner – the reverse is likely to be true. Any discussion regarding investigation and management should start with the simple and practical issues, e.g. a full blood count, chest X-ray, and quickly work through to the more sophisticated and elaborate investigations/treatments. However, when there is one specific diagnostic test which will give the diagnosis, say it straight away. For example, in a case of spastic paraparesis in a young woman with nystagmus and optic neuritis, say you wish to do an MRI of the brain and brainstem, not a full blood count. Do not use abbreviations, e.g. TPR and BP, U+E etc. – although we all use them in our daily work. It is preferable to use the full term in the exam. If you do not understand what the examiner is getting at, ask them politely to repeat the question. This is perfectly acceptable and much better than launching into an inappropriate answer.

Communication skills and ethics (Station 4)

The communication skills and ethics' station aims to assess the ability of the candidate to guide and organise an interview with the subject in a clear and structured manner, provide emotional support and discuss further management issues. There are no marks specifically awarded for medical knowledge, and the ability of the candidate to discuss issues in an open and non-prejudiced manner, rather than simply imparting information, is of paramount importance.

The written instructions will provide a framework for the start of the consultation, but its subsequent direction will depend on your interaction with the patient. The consultation should ideally start with relatively 'open' questions before focusing on specific points with 'closed' questions. It is important to assess the patient's knowledge and expectations of their condition before imparting new information, and patients should be allowed sufficient time to digest information and to ask any questions. Examiners will field questions ranging from, 'How do you think you did?', 'What did you do well or badly?', 'What do you think the patient will remember from the consultation?', to more detailed questions regarding legal issues, e.g. 'How long after a fit can you start driving again?'

As one-third of the allocated marks are for legal and ethical issues, it is vital to consider these during the 5 minutes of preparation at the beginning. These are discussed in detail in the relevant section in the book.

Finally, as always, practise your technique with colleagues – many people make the mistake of failing to prepare for this important part of the exam.

ABOUT THIS BOOK

The PACES exam potentially covers an enormous range of clinical cases and topics. As such it is almost impossible to know every permutation and combination that the examiners may throw at you. The secret to success is to have a thorough basic knowledge of clinical examination and communication skills, which can then be applied to almost any situation you will encounter. Experience has shown that in all three areas of the exam, a number of scenarios are tested time and time again. Practice in these will certainly give you a strong foundation for passing the exam. This book is divided into the same five sections as PACES. Each section begins with guidance on generic skills applicable to that particular area, before covering the essential cases commonly encountered by candidates. It is to be expected that once proficient in all these skills and cases, you are unlikely to be surprised in the exam.

THE CASES AND SCENARIOS

Not all the cases are laid out exactly the same, but the broad pattern is outlined here. We have endeavoured to provide information about the cases not only from the point of view of eliciting the relevant clinical signs on examination, but also to consider the aetiology, differential diagnosis, symptoms, investigations and management.

This renders the book ideally suited for PACES, where one may be asked to examine a patient with hemiparesis; take a history from them; perhaps explain to them what is the likely cause and differential diagnosis; or, finally, to convey information about the outlook and prognosis to them or their family. Thus these are not cases solely to be examined but to be transferred and considered for each station in the examination.

In exactly the same frame of mind, the history-taking scenarios can often be turned round to communication scenarios – again consider the legal and ethical issues around each case as they arise. Think what information you might gather from examining this patient.

Hopefully, after reading this book, candidates will realise that the list of things to know in order to pass the exam is not endless. When you go into the exam you will be at the peak of your ability. The signs will be simple to elicit and the examiners will be impressed not only with your technique but your manner towards the patient. The patients will want you as their doctor and the relatives will never have spoken to someone so understanding, authoritative yet approachable.

Good luck – but you should not need it.

"In critical and baffling situations, it is always best to return to first principle and simple action."

Winston Churchill

STATION 1

The Respiratory and Abdominal Examinations

The Respiratory Examination

In PACES, the majority of respiratory cases will involve chronic conditions that can be identified before auscultation. Therefore it is important to practise one's skills of observation, both of the patient and of the surrounding environment. As the chest is a relatively symmetrical structure, a careful inspection will usually reveal the side of the pathology.

APPROACH TO THE PATIENT

- Introduce yourself to the patient.
- Ask if the patient has any pain.
- Position the patient correctly (sitting up at 45°).
- Expose the chest, completely if possible.
- Explain what you are going to do, 'I would like to examine your chest and lungs, if that is all right with you?'

OBSERVATION

- Observation alone will usually give clues to the origin of the pathological process.
- Look carefully around the bed for oxygen cylinders, inhalers, nebulisers, peak-flow machines, steroid cards or sputum pots.
- Look at the patient – cyanosis, surgical scars (pneumonectomy), steroids, failure to thrive (cystic fibrosis), cachexia (malignancy), productive cough (bronchiectasis), rashes (autoimmune disease and sarcoidosis) or arthropathy (rheumatoid arthritis).
- Stand at the end of the bed, with the patient undressed, and watch the patient breathe. Note the respiratory rate, and the length of the inspiratory and expiratory phase of respiration. Inspiration is usually longer than expiration; this is reversed in emphysema (see p. 21).
- Ask the patient to take a deep breath in and out and look carefully for asymmetry.

Noting the presence of asymmetry at this stage immediately gives you an advantage.

One knows there is likely to be unilateral pathology on the side with reduced ventilation, e.g. pleural effusion, consolidation, collapse or pneumonectomy.

If symmetry is maintained consider pulmonary fibrosis, bronchiectasis or airways disease.

Hands

Look for:
- Tar stains – airways disease and malignancy
- Clubbing – idiopathic, fibrosis, malignancy and bronchiectasis
- Clubbing and swelling of the wrist – hypertrophic pulmonary osteoarthropathy (a rare paraneoplastic manifestation of lung cancer, with classic X-ray changes)
- Cyanosis – central or peripheral
- Tremor – β-agonist therapy
- Flap – dorsiflexed wrists and fingers spread out (carbon dioxide retention).

Pulse

- Bounding – carbon dioxide retention
- Tachycardia – infection and β-agonist therapy

Face

- Conjunctival pallor
- Meiosis – Horner's syndrome
- Lips/tongue – central cyanosis

Neck

- Lymphadenopathy
- Jugular venous pressure (JVP) elevated with 'v' waves – right ventricular failure (cor pulmonale); if suspected, examine for left parasternal (right ventricular) heave and tricuspid regurgitation

INSPECTION OF THE CHEST

Shape of the chest

- Barrel – an increase in the anteroposterior diameter (emphysema)
- Pigeon chest (pectus carinatum) – outward bowing of the sternum (chronic childhood respiratory illness or rickets)
- Funnel chest (pectus excavatum) – developmental defect with depression of the sternum
- Kyphoscoliosis – idiopathic or secondary to polio

Trachea

- Place your index and ring fingers on the sternal notch.
- Place your middle finger on the trachea. It should rest equidistant from the index and ring fingers if the trachea is central. The trachea may be slightly deviated to the right in normal people due to the straightness of the right main bronchus.

Causes of tracheal displacement

- Towards the lesion – upper lobe collapse, fibrosis or pneumonectomy/lobectomy
- Away from the lesion – large pleural effusion or tension pneumothorax

Cardiac apex

- Displaced by pleural effusion/pneumothorax, although may be impalpable
- Also difficult to feel in patients with hyperexpanded chest
- Pulled towards side of collapse/pneumonectomy

The chest

- It may seem obvious that either the front or the back of the chest should be examined completely before proceeding to the other side. A full respiratory examination is quite tiring, especially with respiratory pathology, and thus the patient should not be moved unnecessarily.

PALPATION

- Palpate any deformity or lump.

Expansion

- Assess the upper and lower chest separately.
- Upper chest – place your hands lightly on the patient's upper chest just below the clavicles. You should feel your hands rise anteriorly. Feel for any asymmetry.
- Lower chest – place your hands on the lateral side of the lower ribs, with your thumbs pointing towards the midline. The thumbs may touch lightly in the midline, but this will depend on the size of your hands and the patient's chest. The thumbs should move symmetrically apart during inspiration. Normal expansion is 4–5 cm.

PERCUSSION

- Percuss the clavicles and then the lung fields. Compare left with right at each point, moving down the chest. Do not forget to specifically percuss in each axilla: it is the only place where the upper, middle (lingula on the left) and lower lobes can be examined together.

Tactile Vocal Fremitus (TVF)

- Assess fremitus by asking the patient to say '99' whilst placing the border of your little fingers on the patient's chest wall. Compare the left and right lungs simultaneously by using both hands; move down the chest wall from the top to the bottom.

AUSCULTATION

- Once again move down in a zig-zag manner, asking the patient to breathe quietly through the mouth. Use the diaphragm of the stethoscope on the chest wall, but the bell for the supraclavicular area as it is smaller.

Breath sounds

You should be familiar with the following terms:
- Normal, i.e. vesicular
- Bronchial – noise transmitted to the chest wall from a large airway, e.g. consolidation or along the top of an effusion
- Decreased, e.g. emphysema
- Wheeze – always expiratory: mono/polyphonic
- Stridor – always inspiratory, and indicates extrathoracic obstruction
- Crackles – fine/coarse; inspiratory/expiratory
- Pleural rub – pleurisy secondary to a pulmonary embolus or pneumonia.

Vocal Resonance (VR)

- Analogous to TVF, and can be performed as an alternative. One hears bronchophony over consolidation or fibrosis as well as at the top of an effusion, because the large airways noise is transmitted directly to the chest wall. It sounds as if the words are spoken directly into one's ear. However, it does provide additional information vis-à-vis bleating aegophony and whispering pectoriloquy above an effusion.

Summary of clinical findings in common respiratory cases

	Collapse, local fibrosis, pneumo-nectomy	Consoli-dation	Effusion	Chronic obstructive pulmonary disease (COPD)	Pneumo-thorax (large)	Bilateral fibrosis
Trachea	Deviated towards lesion	No change	No change, deviated away if very large	No change	Usually central, may be deviated away	No change
Expansion	Reduced unilaterally	Reduced unilaterally	Reduced unilaterally	Reduced bilaterally (hyper-expanded)	Reduced unilaterally	No change
Percussion	Dull	Dull	Stony dull	No change	Hyper-resonant	No change
TVF/VR	Reduced	Increased	Reduced (aegophony above)	No change	Reduced	No change
Breath sounds	Quiet	Bronchial breathing	Absent/ reduced	Variable; Quiet ± wheeze	Absent/ reduced	Fine end-inspiratory crackles

TO FINISH

- Measure peak expiratory flow rate.
- Examine any sputum in a pot – quantity, colour (and, traditionally, smell).
- Thank the patient and help them dress.

STATION

Respiratory Scenarios

1. Fibrosing alveolitis
2. Pleural effusion
3. Bronchiectasis
4. Unilateral pulmonary fibrosis
5. Chronic airways disease
6. Lung cancer

1. FIBROSING ALVEOLITIS

Points in the examination

- Evidence of treatment – oxygen cylinder, steroid use
- Finger clubbing
- Central cyanosis
- Fine end-inspiratory basal crepitations/crackles
- Complications – cor pulmonale (right ventricular heave, raised JVP, prominent 'v' waves, peripheral oedema)

Conditions associated with cryptogenic fibrosing alveolitis (CFA)

- Autoimmune hepatitis – cirrhosis ± hepatomegaly
- Sjögren's syndrome – dry eyes and mouth

Other conditions associated with fibrosing alveolitis (not CFA)

- Rheumatoid arthritis – deforming arthropathy (Caplan's syndrome is fibrosing alveolitis associated with exposure to coal dust in patients who tend to be rheumatoid factor-positive)
- Systemic sclerosis – typical appearance of the hands and face, telangiectasia
- Dermatomyositis – heliotrope rash, Gottren's patches and proximal myopathy
- Sarcoidosis – lupus pernio and erythema nodosum
- Pneumoconiosis – asbestosis, silicosis, berylliosis and coal dust
- Extrinsic allergic alveolitis – e.g. bird fancier's or farmer's lung
- Radiation exposure
- Drugs – e.g. amiodarone, bleomycin

Symptoms

- Progressive dyspnoea with chronic unproductive cough
- Arthritis
- Rash

Investigations

- Chest X-ray (CXR) – reticulonodular shadowing, 'honeycomb lung', reduced lung volumes, pleural plaques – asbestosis, bilateral hilar lymphadenopathy (BHL), joint changes in shoulders, dilated oesophagus
- Arterial blood gases – desaturation on exercise
- Respiratory function tests – restrictive defect with decreased gas transfer
- High-resolution computed tomography (CT) – sensitive; can detect fibrosis in the presence of a normal CXR
- Bronchoscopy and bronchoalveolar lavage – increased cells (lymphocytes carry a better prognosis than other cells)
- Open lung biopsy – transbronchial or percutaneous biopsy may be required for histology
- Serum precipitins and full blood count (FBC) (eosinophilia) for extrinsic allergic alveolitis
- Angiotensin-converting enzyme (ACE) levels and autoantibodies

Management

- Oral steroids may provide benefit: those patients who respond have a 60% 5-year survival rate – reduces to only 25% in non-responders.
- Non-responders can be treated with cyclophosphamide.
- Give supplemental oxygen.
- Lung transplantation is an option in younger patients, with rapidly progressive disease there is a 60% 1-year survival rate.
- Patients should be regularly followed up with CXRs and respiratory function tests.

Points of interest

- Hamman–Rich syndrome is an acute form of CFA that responds to steroids, but overall has a poor outcome.
- Pneumoconioses.
  - Silicosis – upper-zone fibrosis, with eggshell hilar calcification that predisposes to TB infection.
  - Berylliosis – granulomatous lesions resulting in fibrosis, similar to sarcoid.
  - Asbestosis – predominantly affects lung bases; pleural plaques and associated mesothelioma.
  - Simple coal-worker's lung does not cause pulmonary fibrosis.

- Sarcoidosis – a multisystem granulomatous disorder characterised by overactivated T lymphocytes:
  - Skin – erythema nodosum, lupus pernio
  - Lungs – bilateral hilar lymphadenopathy, pulmonary nodules and fibrosis
  - Lymphadenopathy, arthropathy and neuropathy
  - Investigations – CXR, serum ACE levels, tissue biopsy (Kveim test is outdated), gallium citrate scan may identify granulomatous disease.
- Extrinsic allergic alveolitis:
  - Bird fancier's lung – pigeons
  - Farmer's lung – mouldy hay
  - Byssinosis – cotton dust
  - Following exposure there is inflammation of the bronchioles resulting in cough, pyrexia and malaise. If exposure becomes chronic it may result in increasing shortness of breath and non-caseating granulomatous disease
  - Treatment is with steroids in acute disease and long-term avoidance of precipitating factors.

2. PLEURAL EFFUSION

Points in the examination

- Tachypnoeic
- Central trachea – a large effusion may push it away
- Apex – impalpable with left-sided effusion, or displaced if on the contralateral side
- Expansion – decreased on the affected side
- Percussion – stony dull on the affected side
- Tactile fremitus or vocal resonance – decreased on the affected side
- Breath sounds – diminished on the affected side
- There may be whispering pectoriloquy ± bronchial breathing above the effusion
- 'Bleating aegophany' may be heard above the level of the effusion.

Clues to the cause

- Malignancy – clubbing, tar-staining, cachexia, Horner's syndrome and lymphadenopathy
- Mastectomy, colostomy or laparotomy, radiation scars and tattoos
- Chemotherapy – alopecia, mucositis, Cushing's syndrome, radiation scars, tuberculosis (TB)/lymphoma – lymphadenopathy and fever
- Pneumonia – purulent sputum, tachypnoea, fever
- Cardiac failure – raised JVP, third heart sound, peripheral oedema
- Nephrotic syndrome – generalised oedema and ascites
- Cirrhosis
- Autoimmune disease – characteristic rash or arthritis
- Pulmonary emboli – raised JVP, right ventricular heave, loud P_2, deep vein thrombosis (DVT)
- Hypothyroidism – dry skin, bradycardia, characteristic facies, slow-relaxing reflexes

Aetiology

- Exudates – protein content >30 g/l:
  - Malignancy – primary, e.g. bronchogenic, mesothelioma, or secondary; infection; pulmonary emboli; connective tissue disease, e.g. rheumatoid arthritis and systemic lupus erythematosus (SLE)
- Transudate – protein content <30 g/l:
  - Heart failure, cirrhosis, nephrotic syndrome, hypothyroidism

Differential diagnosis

- Lung collapse – trachea pulled to affected side, percussion note is not stony dull
- Raised hemidiaphragm:
  - Phrenic nerve palsy, e.g. cancer, motor neurone disease
  - Hepatomegaly – the area of dullness moves with respiration, unlike the former

Symptoms

- Dyspnoea
- Weight loss and lethargy – malignancy
- Productive cough and fever – infection
- Haemoptysis – malignancy, pulmonary emboli and TB
- Arthritis and rash – autoimmune disease
- Abrupt orthopnoea – phrenic nerve palsy

Investigations

- CXR
- Aspiration – protein level, microscopy, culture and sensitivity (MC+S) (including acid-fast bacilli (AFBs)) and cytology
- Pleural biopsy is often required in patients with TB and malignancy
- Sputum MC+S and cytology
- Mantoux test
- Echocardiography
- Thyroid-stimulating hormone (TSH) and thyroxine (T_4) levels
- Antinuclear antibody (ANA), rheumatoid factor, complement C3, C4
- Spiral CT and/or ventilation-perfusion (VQ) scan for pulmonary emboli
- Bronchoscopy ± CT-guided biopsy for tissue diagnosis

Management

- Symptomatic malignant effusions require drainage ± pleurodesis (NB. tube drainage should be avoided in patients with mesothelioma due to risk of seeding).
- Treat underlying cause.

Points of interest

- The incidence of mesothelioma is increasing worldwide due to previous exposure to asbestos; lag phase is 20–40 years. The disease is unresponsive to conventional therapy and prognosis is poor.

Causes of effusion

Exudate	Transudate
Malignancy:	Cardiac failure
– primary (bronchogenic and mesothelioma)	Nephrotic syndrome
– secondary	Cirrhosis
TB	Peritoneal dialysis
Pneumonia	Hypothyroidism
Autoimmune diseases (RA, SLE)	Meigs' syndrome
Pulmonary embolus	
Dressler's syndrome	
Yellow-nail syndrome	
Pancreatitis	

3. BRONCHIECTASIS

Points in the examination

- Clubbing
- Central cyanosis
- Dyspnoeic – increased respiratory rate
- Cachexia and short stature
- Cough with copious purulent sputum (often bloody) and halitosis
- Coarse inspiratory crepitations, often over one or more areas of the lungs

Complications

- Anaemia, brain abscess, cor pulmonale, amyloid

Aetiology

- Childhood infection – whooping cough, measles, TB
- Cystic fibrosis – young, cachectic, short stature
- Kartagener's syndrome – dextrocardia, azoospermia
- Bronchial obstruction – malignancy, TB, lymph nodes
- Hypogammaglobulinaemia (congenital and acquired)
- Allergic bronchopulmonary aspergillosis

Symptoms

- Childhood chest infections
- Previous TB
- Infertility
- Cystic fibrosis – failure to thrive, gastrointestinal symptoms

Investigations

- FBC
- Sputum MC+S
- CXR
- High-resolution CT of chest
- Sweat test

- Serum immunoglobulins – decreased IgA in hypogammaglobulinaemia
- Mantoux test
- Biopsy

Treatment

- Postural drainage
- Antibiotics – cover *Pseudomonas* spp.
- Bronchodilators and steroids – if any reversible component
- Mucolytics – nebulised rhDNase is effective in patients with viscid sputum
- Surgery for localised disease
- Gene therapy – for cystic fibrosis

Points of interest

- Cystic fibrosis (CF) – autosomal recessive disease, chromosome 7, mutation is present in 1/25 patients; thus homozygosity in 1/2,500. The ΔF_{508} mutation is present in 70% of patients and is associated with a poorer prognosis.
  - Presentation:
    - meconium ileus – in infants
    - malabsorption/failure to thrive – in children
    - bronchiectasis – as teenagers
    - diabetes develops in 20% of adults due to destruction of the islets of Langerhans by mucoid plugging of the pancreatic ducts
    - diagnosis is by sweat-testing, (sweat chloride >60 mmol/l); patients and families should be counselled before testing; genetic testing is helpful for prognosis.
- In the past, survival has not usually been beyond the third decade of life. Improved antibiotics, immunisation against *Pseudomonas* spp., aggressive postural drainage, aerosolised rhDNase and gene therapy have resulted in increased overall survival for these patients, to their fourth decade. Gene therapy comprises inhaled transfer of the wild-type cystic fibrosis transmembrane conductor regulator (CFTR) gene, using either a liposomal or viral vector, to the bronchial mucosa.
- Men are infertile. Pregnant women with a family history can undergo chorionic villus sampling.

4. UNILATERAL PULMONARY FIBROSIS

Points in the examination

- Trachea – deviated towards lesion if involving the upper lobes
- Radiotherapy marks
- Thoracotomy scar
- Rib resection ± supraclavicular scar (old TB)
- Expansion – decreased on affected side
- Percussion – dullness on affected side
- Tactile vocal fremitus and vocal resonance – increased on affected side
- Coarse inspiratory and expiratory crackles

Aetiology of upper lobe fibrosis

- Treated tuberculosis – thoracotomy and rib resection with iatrogenic lobar collapse. A supraclavicular scar may indicate prior phrenic nerve crush. Both these procedures will have rendered the lung hypoxic and thus had an antituberculous effect prior to effective chemotherapy.
- Malignant disease – clubbing, thoracotomy, radiotherapy marks, lymphadenopathy, hepatomegaly, Horner's syndrome, wasting of the small muscles of the hand (Pancoast's tumour).

Differential diagnosis

- Lobar pneumonia – associated with pyrexia, but it is an unlikely examination case
- Bronchiectasis – productive cough, clubbing

Symptoms

- With old TB the patient may be asymptomatic; as the lung volume is decreased, dyspnoea may occur with exertion – rest and home oxygen if respiratory failure occurs.
- With reactivation of TB there may be constitutional symptoms – weight loss, fever, night sweats.
- Malignancy – may be accompanied by weight loss, cough/haemoptysis, chest pain, lymphadenopathy, wasting of the small muscles of the hand.

Investigations

- CXR
- FBC
- Urea and electrolytes
- Erythrocyte sedimentation rate (ESR), C-reactive protein (CRP)
- Sputum cytology, smear and culture – if active infection suspected; smear-positive TB warrants isolation
- High-resolution CT

Management

- If asymptomatic, with unilateral fibrosis – no treatment is required.
- If active TB is suspected – investigate and treat along standard lines (see pp. 108–111).
- If malignancy is suspected – arrange a tissue biopsy and staging.

5. CHRONIC AIRWAYS DISEASE

Chronic bronchitis and emphysema are two separate diseases that usually coexist, although patients tend to suffer from one predominantly. Bronchitis is a clinical diagnosis relating to chronic cough and sputum production, while emphysema is a pathological diagnosis characterised by dilatation of the terminal air spaces. The two diseases are usually described as a single entity – chronic airways disease (CAL (chronic airflow limitation), COAD (chronic obstructive airways disease), or COPD (chronic obstructive pulmonary disease)).

Points in the examination

- Signs of treatment:
  - Cushingoid appearance, ecchymoses, fine tremor (β_2-agonist), inhalers, nebulisers and oxygen mask/cylinders

Clinical signs favouring chronic bronchitis ('blue bloaters')

- Central cyanosis
- Bounding pulse, coarse flapping tremor
- Barrel chest, often moderately obese
- Cough and sputum production
- Wheeze and crackles in the chest – widespread

Clinical signs favouring emphysema ('pink puffers')

- Tachypnoea
- Hyperinflated chest; patients are often thin
- Reduced suprasternal notch–cricoid cartilage distance
- Decreased chest movement and increased use of accessory muscles
- Hyper-resonance
- Decreased breath sounds – particularly over bullae
- Prolonged expiration and pursed lips – to maintain pressure in the lungs and prevent airway collapse (effectively, this is positive end-expiratory airways pressure, PEEP)

Associated conditions

- Pneumonia – increased dyspnoea, pyrexia, change in sputum colour, dullness to percussion with increased TVF, crepitations and bronchial breathing over infected area
- Lung cancer – Horner's syndrome, cachexia, anaemia, lymphadenopathy
- Pulmonary hypertension leading to cor pulmonale – raised JVP 'cv' waves, peripheral oedema, left parasternal heave, palpable 2nd heart sound, and tricuspid regurgitation (TR)

Aetiology

- Cigarette smoking
- Atmospheric pollution
- α_1-antitrypsin deficiency (emphysema) – predominantly affects the upper lobes

Points in the history

- Multiple exacerbations
- Details of previous admissions – including to an intensive therapy unit (ITU) – and treatment, particularly steroids
- Previous arterial blood gases
- Current treatment
- Dyspnoea and cough
- What is the precipitating factor in this case?
- Calculate the number of pack-years smoked.

Investigations

- FBC, urea and electrolytes
- CXR
- Arterial blood gases
- Blood and sputum culture
- ECG
- Lung function tests
- α_1-antitrypsin levels

Management

- Oxygen (24% until dependence on hypoxic drive is established)
- Nebulised β_2-agonists, antimuscarinics and steroids (inhaled and oral) if the disease has a reversible component – requires lung function tests
- Aminophylline
- Antibiotics, if infective component
- Newer treatments:
  - Leukotriene β_4-agonists
  - Interleukin-8 antagonists
  - Tumour necrosis factor (TNF) inhibitors

Points of interest

- External artificial ventilation:
  - CPAP – continuous positive airway pressure ventilation, used in individuals with healthy lungs who require artificial support; it is also used for obstructive sleep apnoea, as it maintains open airways
  - NIPPV – nasal intermittent positive pressure ventilation; used for patients with neuromuscular deficits, e.g. polio, or in CO_2 retainers; ventilation is triggered by inspiration
  - BIPAP – bilevel positive airway pressure ventilation; used for patients with underlying airway disease; the positive pressure keeps the airways open, allowing oxygen transfer
- Indications for domiciliary oxygen
  - Stable disease
  - FEV_1 <1.5 litres; FVC <2 litres (FEV_1, forced expiratory volume in 1 second; FVC, forced vital capacity)
  - *PaO*$_2$ (partial arterial pressure of oxygen) <7.3 kPa
  - Non-smoking – explosion risk

6. LUNG CANCER

Points in the examination

- Clubbing and tar-stained fingers
- Thoracotomy scar from surgical removal of primary tumour ± radiotherapy marks
- Cachexia
- Supraclavicular/cervical lymphadenopathy
- Pleural effusion (see p. 14)
- Unilateral collapse and fibrosis (see p. 19)

Associations with lung cancer

Local effects

- Superior vena cava obstruction – facial oedema, fixed dilatation of superficial neck veins, suffusion and often stridor
- Horner's syndrome and wasting of the small muscles of the hand, Pancoast's tumour (see also p. 19)
- Recurrent laryngeal nerve palsy – hoarse voice

Metastatic effects

- Spinal cord compression
- Focal neurology – brain metastases, especially small-cell lung cancer
- Hepatomegaly ± jaundice

Paraneoplastic syndromes

Neurological

- Peripheral neuropathy
- Cerebellar signs
- Eaton–Lambert syndrome – proximal muscle weakness and fatigue; it is similar to myasthenia gravis, except that power is often improved after brief exercise and reflexes are restored soon after activity

Endocrine

- Ectopic ACTH production – pigmentation Cushing's syndrome – small-cell carcinoma
- Parathyroid hormone-related peptide production hypercalcaemia – usually by squamous-cell carcinoma
- Syndrome of inappropriate antidiuretic hormone (secretion) (SIADH) – confusion, nausea, vomiting

Dermatological/rheumatological

- Dermatomyositis (p. 355)
- Clubbing
- Hypertrophic pulmonary osteoarthropathy

Other

- Recurrent venous thrombosis
- Pericarditis
- Marantic endocarditis

Aetiology

- Cigarette smoking
- Manufacturing – asbestosis, chromate, nickel, arsenic
- Radioactivity – uranium mining

Symptoms

- Cough, haemoptysis, breathlessness, hoarseness
- Weight loss, malaise
- Chest pain, lymphadenopathy
- Related to metastatic/paraneoplastic effects

Initial investigations

- CXR
- Sputum cytology
- Bronchoscopy and biopsy
- Pleural aspiration and biopsy – if effusion present

Further investigations (staging)

- Ultrasound of liver
- CT thorax (hilar lymphadenopathy), liver, adrenals
- Liver function tests (LFTs), bone profile
- Pulmonary function tests
- Bone scan
- Positron-emission tomography (PET) scan useful for mediastinal disease

Management

- Surgery – rarely suitable, due to frequent local spread. Requires adequate lung function (FEV_1 >1.2 litres for lobectomy, >1.5 litres for pneumonectomy)
- Chemotherapy – for small-cell cancer, although prognosis remains poor
- Radiotherapy – useful for palliative relief of haemoptysis and bony pain
- Endobronchial laser – palliative treatment of local bronchial obstruction

The Abdominal Examination

The majority of cases will be associated with patterns of organomegaly. However, there are many peripheral signs to be uncovered. With 10 minutes to perform a thorough examination and to discuss one's findings, time can still be tight. Although the key part of the examination is the abdomen itself, the search for peripheral signs, which are legion, must be accomplished rapidly yet thoroughly. They will often give clues as to the main pathology. In PACES, the majority of patients will fall into one of three main patterns of pathology:

- Liver disease (primary or secondary) – cirrhosis, portal hypertension, encephalopathy; or associated with heart failure, metastatic disease, infective agents, infiltration or inflammation
- Splenomegaly or hepatosplenomegaly – myeloproliferative, lymphoproliferative or autoimmune disease
- Renal disease ± evidence of renal replacement.

APPROACH TO THE PATIENT

- Introduction – introduce yourself to the patient by name.
- Ask the patient if he/she has any pain.
- Position the patient correctly – lying flat, with the head resting on one pillow. The abdomen should be relaxed with the arms by their sides.
- Expose the patient from the groin upwards. Full inspection must include the external genitalia, but, for the purpose of the exam and for the modesty of the patients, it is prudent to expose only down to the pubic tubercle. Similarly, the breasts can remain covered in ladies.
- Explain what you are going to do: 'I am just going to feel your tummy, if that's all right' will usually suffice.

INSPECTION

General observation

- Ask yourself which of the three groups mentioned above the patient is likely to fall into.
- Stand at the end of the bed and take time looking at the patient. Ask the patient to take a deep breath in and look carefully for descending masses, e.g. liver, spleen or kidneys.
- Look for the following additional clues as to the origin of the disease:
  - Splenomegaly or hepatosplenomegaly:
    - lymphadenopathy
    - bruises and pallor
  - Renal disease:
    - nephrectomy scar or renal transplant scar in the iliac fossa
    - previous chronic ambulatory peritoneal dialysis scars or arteriovenous fistulas
    - cushingoid appearance
  - Primary liver disease:
    - jaundice or scratch marks
    - spider naevi – occur in drainage site of superior vena cava; more than 4 or 5 is probably abnormal; they are fed by a central arteriole and can be obliterated by pressure over the arteriole
    - abdominal distension – ascites
    - tattoos, or needle tracks from intravenous drug use – hepatitis B
    - vitiligo or arthropathy – autoimmune disease
    - gynaecomastia and loss of secondary sexual hair
  - Secondary liver disease:
    - cachexia – malignancy
    - dyspnoea, peripheral oedema, raised JVP – heart failure
    - bronzing or slate-grey skin – haemochromatosis
    - lupus pernio – sarcoidosis.

Now proceed to a more detailed examination.

Nails and hands

- Leuconychia, koilonychia, clubbing or cyanosis
- Nail-fold infarcts – vasculitis
- Blotchy palmar erythema (liver palms)
- Dupuytren's contracture
- Asterixis (a coarse flap becoming apparent after a few seconds with the arms and wrists extended)

Skin

- Purpura and bruises; skin thickness (thin in Cushing's syndrome)
- Xanthomas – commonly seen in primary biliary cirrhosis
- Also Kaposi's sarcoma in AIDS; erythema nodosum in sarcoid, Crohn's disease or ulcerative colitis; pyoderma gangrenosum in inflammatory bowel disease; radiation marks
- Tattoos
- Pallor
- Icterus
- Uveitis – autoimmune or inflammatory bowel disease
- Kayser–Fleischer rings in Descemet's membrane – best seen with a slit lamp in Wilson's disease
- Cheilosis – iron, folate, vitamin B_{12} or B_6 deficiency
- Oral ulcers – inflammatory bowel or coeliac disease; extragenital syphilis; Behçet's disease
- Leucoplakia or oral herpes – AIDS
- Pigmentation – drugs, Addison's disease, Peutz–Jeghers' syndrome (autosomal dominant condition with brown spots on the lips, oral mucosa, around the mouth, face and occasionally elsewhere on the skin; associated with hamartomatous polyps of the small and large bowel which only rarely become malignant)
- Tongue – smooth and red in vitamin B_{12} deficiency, geographical tongue (can occur in riboflavin/vitamin B_2 deficiency)
- Telangiectasia – hereditary haemorrhagic telangiectasia (Osler–Weber–Rendu syndrome – autosomal dominant condition with mucosal telangiectasia; presents with gastrointestinal bleeding or epistaxis. The telangiectasia also occur in the retina and brain)
- Gums – hypertrophy with phenytoin, ciclosporin and acute myeloid leukaemia (AML)
- Teeth – real or false, and their condition
- Breath – fetor hepaticus in the late stages of liver disease is a sweet smell; uraemia produces a fishy, ammoniacal smell
- Parotids – enlarged in alcoholics, sarcoid, anorexia and Sjögren's syndrome. Unilateral parotid enlargement is usually associated with a blocked duct or tumour and often accompanied by a facial nerve palsy.

Neck and chest

- Lymphadenopathy – enlargement of Virchow's node in the left supraclavicular fossa is Troissier's sign, classically, but not exclusively, seen in advanced gastric carcinoma. As well as the neck, examine the nodes in the axillas, epitrochlear, para-aortic, inguinal, femoral and popliteal regions.
- As it is best to examine lymph nodes in the neck from behind, now is the opportunity to examine the patient's back for spider naevi, scars, tattoos, etc.
- Gynaecomastia – palpate the subcutaneous breast tissue bilaterally.
- Loss of axillary hair.

Abdomen

- Observe the abdomen carefully, asking the patient to take a deep breath in. Do not be afraid to spend a moment or two properly inspecting the abdomen – if needs be by kneeling at the patient's side, as well as from the end of the bed. Look specifically for the liver or spleen moving down, fullness in the flanks and distension.
- Corkscrew hairs with perifollicular haemorrhage are frequently seen in alcoholics with vitamin C deficiency, along with gingivitis.
- Stretch marks – atrophic and silvery indicate previous distension – usually striae gravidarum, occasionally drained ascites – or purple and livid in Cushing's syndrome.
- Prominent superficial veins can be seen in three situations:
  - Thin veins over the costal margin – in normal people
  - Caput medusae in portal hypertension; flow away from the umbilicus.
  - Obstruction of the inferior vena cava; flow towards the head
  From the above details it can be seen that determining the flow in a vein below the umbilicus will delineate the cause, and differentiate between portal hypertension and inferior vena cava (IVC) obstruction.

PALPATION

- The abdomen is divided into nine regions by two horizontal lines (under the inferior costal margin and above the anterior superior iliac spines) and two vertical lines (in the mid-clavicular lines).
- Palpation should be performed from a kneeling position.

- Look at the patient and not your hand whilst palpating to ensure you are causing no discomfort.
- The forearm and hand are held in the same plane, i.e. the wrist is not extended. The pulps of the fingers rather than the tips are used, with slight flexion at the metacarpophalangeal joints to mould to the abdominal wall. The hands may need to be warmed.
- Palpate lightly and quickly the nine regions in turn to determine if there are obvious masses or organomegaly. Avoid any areas of pain till last.
- Now use deeper palpation in each region in turn.

Palpating the liver

- Start from the right iliac fossa and move vertically upwards to the right subcostal region using the sensitive radial border of the index finger to detect any liver enlargement.
- Ask the patient to take deep breaths in as you palpate. During inspiration, as the liver descends, press the fingers inwards and up.
- During expiration, advance your hand 1–2 cm towards the costal margin and repeat the procedure.
- If the liver is felt, ascertain the following:
  - Soft (normal), firm (inflamed or infiltrated) or hard (advanced cirrhosis or metastases)?
  - Smooth or nodular – if nodular, micronodular or macronodular?
  - Pulsatile? – tricuspid regurgitation
  - Tender? – TR, Budd–Chiari syndrome, hepatitis, hepatocellular cancer, abscess
  - Riedel's lobe (a tongue-like projection from the inferior surface of the right lobe, it can extend to the right iliac fossa)

Palpating the spleen

- Start from the right iliac fossa and move diagonally to the left subcostal region with your right hand.
- Place your left hand behind the left lower ribs and apply sustained pressure anteriorly.
- Once again, ask the patient to take deep breaths. During inspiration, press the radial edge of your hand inwards and upwards in an arc towards the left costal margin, to palpate the splenic edge as it moves down towards the right iliac fossa.

- If uncertainty remains, ask the patient to roll onto the right side facing towards you. Place your left hand under the patient's left ribs while your right hand palpates under the costal margin. The spleen may be tipped in this position.

Palpating the kidneys

- The kidneys are bimanually palpable or ballottable.
- Place your left hand under the patient's flank below the 12th rib, just lateral to the long strap muscles of the spine; place your right hand anteriorly.
- Push your bottom hand upwards, and an enlarged kidney can be felt captured between the hands.
- If this is not possible it may be ballottable, where the kidney can be felt to float towards the anterior hand when the posterior fingers flex quickly at maximal inspiration.
- They descend on inspiration and the right kidney may be palpable in healthy slender individuals.

Distinguishing between a liver/spleen and kidney

- One cannot get above a liver or spleen, i.e. one cannot feel a space between them and the costal margin.
- The spleen has a notch.
- The spleen moves inferomedially on inspiration, whereas the kidney moves inferiorly.
- The liver and spleen are not ballottable unless there is gross ascites present.
- Kidneys often have overlying bowel and are resonant to percussion.
- A friction rub may be heard over a spleen, but never over a kidney as it is too posterior.

Other masses

- The bladder and bowel may be felt in normal individuals. The bladder rises out of the pelvis in the mid-line and pressure may induce a desire to micturate. Faeces in the bowel can be indented by the examining finger, a unique feature.
- The aorta should be palpated for in the mid-line above the umbilicus. The normal diameter is up to 3 cm.
- Pancreatic pseudocysts, if large, can be felt in the epigastric region; they feel fixed and do not descend.

- Other pelvic masses, such as ovarian tumours, a gravid uterus or fibroids, all arise out of the pelvis, the former being eccentrically placed. *Per rectum* or *vaginam* examination is helpful to clarify their nature, but should not be performed in PACES.

PERCUSSION

- Percussion is an art: the more experienced one becomes, the gentler and more refined it is. It is highly discriminatory.
- The abdominal viscera can have thin leading edges that are easily missed by a heavy-handed approach, leading to the observation that, 'The closer one gets to the (Buckingham) Palace, the quieter one's percussion' (Sir Ronald Bodley Scott).

Percussion of the liver and spleen

- The liver and spleen are dull to percussion.
- Percussion should follow a similar pattern to palpation, starting in the right iliac fossa and moving vertically up for the liver and diagonally for the spleen.
- Percussion should continue up the chest to define the upper border of the liver, which should extend beyond the 6th rib. This determines whether the liver is truly enlarged or displaced inferiorly by a hyperexpanded chest or subdiaphragmatic collection.
- In the mid-clavicular line, the liver span should be no greater than 12 cm.
- The lower border of a normal spleen is the 9th rib in the mid-axillary line. Dullness between this surface marking and the costal margin indicates mild splenomegaly. This is the only clinical way of detecting this degree of enlargement.

Percussion for ascites

- Percuss horizontally across the abdomen through the umbilicus. If an area of dullness is found in the left or right flanks, keep the finger in that position. Ask the patient to roll away or towards you so your finger is uppermost and wait for 20 seconds. Percuss again, and if resonant it is indicative of ascites. This is 'shifting dullness'.
- If there are no areas of dullness initially, there is no need to ask the patient to roll to one side, as there is no area of dullness to shift.

- If there is tense ascites one may be able to demonstrate a fluid thrill:
  - Ask either the examiner or patient to place the side of their hand in the mid-line of the abdomen, pressing firmly down.
  - With one hand pressed against the left side of the abdomen flick the near side. A percussion wave felt is the fluid thrill.

AUSCULTATION

- Listen with the diaphragm for up to 30 seconds.
- Bowel sounds cannot be heard in a paralytic ileus or bowel obstruction.
- If one suspects pyloric obstruction or peptic ulcer disease, a succussion splash can be heard.
- Listen to the renal arteries posteriorly, at the sides of the long strap muscles, below the 12th rib, for bruits. Also listen anteriorly in the epigastrium for a bruit in an abdominal aortic aneurysm (AAA), over the femoral arteries for bruits and over an enlarged liver and spleen for bruits (hepatocellular carcinoma) or rubs.

Lastly

- Palpate the hernial orifices.
- Say you would wish to examine the external genitalia and perform a *per rectum* examination.
- Test the patient's urine with a dipstick.
- Thank and cover the patient; sit them up.

Abdominal Scenarios

1. TRANSPLANTED KIDNEY

Points in the examination

- Signs of previous renal replacement therapy (forearm fistula or peritoneal dialysis scars)
- Evidence of immunosuppressive therapy (gum hypertrophy, cushingoid appearance, skin tumours)
- Mass in the iliac fossa, with overlying scar (J-shaped) consistent with transplanted kidney
- Assess graft function – uraemia, shortness of breath, graft tenderness

Aetiology of the renal failure

- Lipodystrophy associated with membranous glomerulonephritis
- Polycystic kidneys in the abdomen
- Signs of diabetes, e.g. glucometer, glucose stix, foot ulcers and poor vision
- Other autoimmune conditions, e.g. SLE (rashes), vitiligo

Differential diagnosis for a mass in the iliac fossa

- Crohn's disease – mouth ulcers, anal disease, abdominal scars, skin rashes
- Primary malignancy (bowel, ovarian) – lymph nodes, hepatomegaly, cachexia
- Iliac TB mass – fever, lymph nodes, evidence of respiratory disease
- Appendicular abscess
- Caecal carcinoid

Causes of endstage renal failure in the UK

- Diabetes
- Glomerulonephritis
- Chronic pyelonephritis
- Polycystic kidneys
- Interstitial nephritis
- Hypertension

Symptoms

- Most patients in the exam will have a transplanted kidney that is functioning well. Symptoms pointing towards graft rejection include tenderness over the graft, fever, hypertension, increased shortness of breath (fluid retention) and decreased urine output.

Investigations

Diagnosis of chronic renal failure (CRF)

- Urea and electrolytes (U+E) – elevated creatinine, acidosis, hyperkalaemia
- FBC – normocytic, normochromic anaemia
- Bone profile – hypocalcaemia, hyperphosphataemia
- 24-h creatinine clearance

Aetiology

- Renal ultrasound – exclude obstruction
- Glucose, HbA1$_c$
- FBC, ESR – autoimmune disease, myeloma
- Urinalysis – proteinuria, red-cell casts, pyuria, cytology
- Antinuclear antibody (ANA), double-stranded (ds)DNA, complement C3/C4, antineutrophil cytoplasmic antibody (ANCA), anti-GBM (glomerular basement membrane), rheumatiod factor (RF) levels
- Serum protein and urine electrophoresis
- Antistreptolysin O (ASO) titre
- Hepatitis B and C serology
- Prostate-specific antigen (PSA)
- Technetium-99m labelled DTPA (diethylenetriamine penta-acetic acid) renogram or MAG3 (mercaptoacetyl triglycine) renogram – gives the percentage contribution of each kidney to the glomerular filtration rate (GFR)
- Renal biopsy

Management of renal transplant patients

- Monitor serum creatinine levels.
- Observe for signs of rejection and secondary malignancy.
- Immunosuppressive drugs (see opposite).
- Address cardiovascular risk factors (major cause of mortality).

Side-effects of immunosuppressive therapy

- Opportunistic infections – e.g. herpes zoster virus, (*Pneumocystis carinii* pneumonia, (PCP), cytomegalovirus (CMV)
- Malignancy – skin, lymphoma
- Ciclosporin – gum hypertrophy, hypertension, nephrotoxicity, CNS disturbance
- Azathioprine – hypersensitivity reactions and bone marrow suppression
- Tacrolimus – similar to ciclosporin, more CNS disturbance
- Glucocorticoids – Cushing's syndrome, osteoporosis, avascular necrosis

Points of interest

- 2,000 transplants take place in the UK every year, with an 80% 5-year success rate for live donors with one matched haplotype. Success rates are lower for cadaver kidneys. HLA-matching improves graft survival and exposes an individual to fewer antigens, thus making a second transplant easier, if required. In contrast, the 5-year survival of a 60-year-old, non-diabetic dialysis patient is approximately 60% (30% for diabetics).
- Rejection is most likely to take place in the first 3 months. Immunosuppressive drugs such as ciclosporin, azathioprine, tacrolimus and glucocorticoids are used. Early signs of rejection include declining renal function and pain, but these can also be due to infection or nephrotoxicity. Many patients will require a biopsy to establish the cause.
- Focal segmental glomerulonephritis can recur in transplanted kidneys. As this results in graft loss in only 15% of affected patients it is not a contraindication to transplantation.

Continuous ambulatory peritoneal dialysis (CAPD)

- The peritoneum acts as the semipermeable membrane; dialysis takes place via a peritoneal catheter. Small abdominal scars remain after removal. Dialysis is required up to three times per day and involves attaching bags to the peritoneal catheter. The main risk is infection. Contraindications include previous abdominal surgery or diverticular disease.

Haemodialysis

- This is performed via a fistula in the forearm; patients often have more than one fistula. Dialysis usually occurs for 3 hours, three times a week in hospital. Satellite dialysis units have improved patient access. An adequate blood pressure and good functioning cardiovascular system are required for haemodialysis as fluid shift is more intense.

CAPD vs. haemodialysis

- CAPD is more flexible and can be performed at home. However, there is a greater risk of infection and the process needs to be performed three times a day.
- Haemodialysis requires more time travelling to a dialysis centre and is less flexible, but gives superior electrolyte control.
- Assessment of dialysis patients:
  - Weight – patients know their 'dry weight'
  - Potassium and ECG changes associated with hyperkalaemia
  - Pulmonary oedema and hypertension.

2. POLYCYSTIC KIDNEY DISEASE

Points in the examination

- Evidence of renal replacement therapy – fistulas in the forearm, catheter scars on the abdomen
- Bilateral or unilateral bimanually palpable mass in the abdomen; often one or both kidneys have been removed, resulting in nephrectomy scars
- Liver cysts causing irregular hepatomegaly
- Kidney transplant:
  - Characteristic J-shaped scar in the iliac fossa
  - Side-effects of immunosuppressive therapy – gum hypertrophy, skin tumours (see p. 39)
- Anaemia is uncommon in these individuals due to the overproduction of erythropoietin
- Neurological deficit – associated berry aneurysms, resulting in subarachnoid haemorrhage in the minority of patients
- Hypertension – ask to measure the blood pressure; is the patient on β-blockers? (bradycardia and cold peripheries)

Differential diagnosis of a renal mass

- Renal cell carcinoma – associated with weight loss, lymphadenopathy and paraneoplastic syndromes (polycythaemia and hypercalcaemia)
- Hydronephrosis
- Adrenal mass – phaeochromocytoma, carcinoma
  (Candidates must be able to distinguish between a renal mass and liver/spleen; see p. 32)

Aetiology

- Polycystic kidney disease is usually autosomal dominant (chromosome 16), although an autosomal recessive form of the disease also occurs (15% of cases). It occurs in 1 in 400–1,000 people. Cysts are invariably present by 18 years of age, and can also occur in the liver, pancreas and spleen. The cysts are easily visible on ultrasound scanning.

Symptoms

- Acute loin pain and/or haematuria
- Abdominal discomfort
- Headaches – sudden onset may be related to subarachnoid haemorrhage
- Symptoms of renal failure occur as renal function declines with time; patients are at increased risk of urinary tract infections (UTIs) and pyelonephritis.

Investigations

- U+E, FBC
- Urinalysis
- Ultrasound
- Intravenous urography (IVU) for hydronephrosis
- Magnetic resonance imaging (MRI) cerebral angiogram – berry aneurysms

Management

- Once the disease is established, patients require regular renal monitoring as 80% of patients have endstage renal failure by their 8th decade; a sudden decline in renal function can occur due to hypertension or pyelonephritis.
- Hypertension should be carefully controlled, as it may result in deterioration of renal function and predispose to an intracranial event.
- Family members should be counselled and screened with ultrasound – cysts can be identified at about 18 years of age. Currently, there is no widely available genetic test.
- A positive family history of subarachnoid haemorrhage requires MRI scanning of the brain, as 20% will have a cerebral aneurysm.

3. SPLENOMEGALY

Points in the examination

- Mass in the left upper quadrant.
- The mass moves diagonally downwards to the right with respiration.
- Unable to palpate above it.
- The presence of a notch.
- Dullness to percussion – the area over the 9th rib at the mid-axillary line should be resonant if the spleen is of normal size.

Other signs associated with splenomegaly

- Lymphadenopathy – myelo/lymphoproliferative disorders, infections and sarcoid
- Purpura and anaemia – myelo/lymphoproliferative disorders
- Rheumatoid arthritis, neutropenia and splenomegaly (Felty's syndrome)
- Signs of chronic liver disease – portal hypertension
- Signs of infection – bacterial endocarditis, sore throat (Epstein–Barr virus, EBV)
- Rashes – e.g. lupus pernio, erythema nodosum (sarcoid); butterfly rash, alopecia areata, vasculitic rash (SLE)

Aetiology

Common causes in the UK

- Malignant causes – lymphoproliferative and myeloproliferative diseases
- Infective causes – EBV-, CMV-, HIV-related opportunistic infections, e.g. *Mycoplasma avium* complex, bacterial endocarditis, malaria and brucellosis
- Autoimmune diseases – SLE, rheumatoid arthritis (Felty's syndrome)
- Portal hypertension of any cause

Rarer causes

- Sarcoid
- Amyloid
- Glycogen storage diseases, e.g. Gaucher's disease
- Autoimmune haemolytic anaemias

Common causes worldwide

- Chronic malaria (falciparum)
- Kala-azar (visceral leishmaniasis)
- Lymphoproliferative and myeloproliferative diseases

Causes of massive splenomegaly

- Chronic malaria
- Chronic myeloid leukaemia (CML)
- Myelofibrosis
- Gaucher's disease

Symptoms of splenomegaly

- Abdominal distension/mass
- Related to underlying cause, e.g.:
  - Lethargy, bleeding – bone marrow failure
  - Drenching night sweats, weight loss and pyrexias (B symptoms) – infections and malignancy
  - Joint pain – Felty's syndrome (rheumatoid arthritis) or SLE
  - Episodes of jaundice – cirrhosis

Initial investigations

- FBC, ESR, blood film
- LFTs
- CXR – lymphoma, sarcoid, TB
- Liver ultrasound
- ANA, Rh F, dsDNA, C3/C4
- Serum ACE
- Blood cultures
- Viral serology – hepatitis, HIV
- Urinalysis – haematuria (endocarditis), proteinuria (myeloma)

Subsequent investigations

- Infections:
  - Thick and thin film, echocardiogram, brucella antibodies
- Lymphoproliferative/myeloproliferative disorders
  - Lymph node biopsy or bone marrow aspirate and trephine
  - Coombs' test (if anaemic)
  - CT chest/abdomen/pelvis for staging of disease
  - Histology, cytogenetics and molecular genetics are essential for classification of haematological malignancy and are of prognostic significance.

Points of interest

- Lymphoproliferative disorders
  - Acute lymphoblastic leukaemia (ALL) – a childhood disease associated with blasts in the blood and bone marrow and good overall survival
  - Chronic lymphatic leukaemia (CLL) – affects elderly patients; lymphadenopathy and pancytopenia more often than splenomegaly
  - Hodgkin's disease – Reed–Sternberg cells, lymphadenopathy, splenomegaly and B symptoms
  - Non-Hodgkin's lymphoma:
    - Low grade – indolent course; but can transform to high grade
    - High grade – aggressive disease; bone marrow and CNS are sometimes involved
  - Hairy-cell leukaemia – associated with 'hairy' cells in the bone marrow and pancytopenia
  - Sézary syndrome (blood correlate of mycosis fungoides) – a form of lymphoma associated with a characteristic skin and lymph node involvement
- Myeloproliferative disorders
  - A series of interrelated diseases which can transform into acute myeloid leukaemia
  - AML – median age 65 years, pancytopenia, gum hypertrophy occurs in M4 and M5 subtypes and disseminated intravascular coagulation is characteristic of the M3 subtype; patients have a relatively poor overall survival
  - CML – median age 45 years, splenomegaly and bone marrow failure; associated with Philadelphia chromosome ($9q^+$, $22q^-$)
  - Myelofibrosis – fibrosis in the bone marrow, resulting in extramedullary haemopoiesis in the liver and spleen

- Polycythaemia rubra vera – moderate splenomegaly, veno-occlusive disease and gout. Good prognosis
- Essential thrombocythaemia

4. HEPATOSPLENOMEGALY

Points in the examination

- The majority of causes of hepatosplenomegaly overlap with those of splenomegaly (see p. 43).
- Mass in right subcostal region descending with respiration.
- Palpable liver enlarged by ...cm below costal margin – note whether smooth/nodular, firm/hard or tender.
- Spleen enlarged by ...cm?
- Both organs are dull to percussion.
- Unable to get above either mass.

Aetiology

- Most causes overlap with splenomegaly, e.g.:
  - Myeloproliferative disorders
  - Lymphoproliferative disorders
  - Amyloid, Gaucher's disease, brucellosis
  - Cirrhosis with portal hypertension.
- Polycystic kidney disease (isolated splenic cysts are very unusual).

Worldwide causes

- Malaria
- Kala-azar

Symptoms

- Abdominal fullness or discomfort
- Constitutional or B symptoms associated with myelo/lymphoproliferative disorders

Investigations

See pp. 44, 45, for *Splenomegaly.*

5. HEPATOMEGALY

Points in the examination

- Palpable mass in the right upper quadrant …cm below the costal margin?
- Consistency – smooth/nodular; firm/hard?
- Moves down with respiration.
- Dull to percussion.
- Unable to palpate above the mass.
- A bruit over the liver is associated with hepatocellular carcinoma.
- ± Signs of chronic liver disease (see p. 28 and 50)

Aetiology

Common causes

- Cardiac failure (± tricuspid regurgitation)
- Viral hepatitis (EBV, CMV, hepatitis A, B and C) – tattoos, intravenous drug use
- Malignancy – cachexia, lymphadenopathy, previous surgery (mastectomy, colostomy), Beau's lines or radiotherapy marks
- Cirrhosis (see p. 50)

Uncommon causes

- Haemochromatosis – skin pigmentation, diabetes, arthropathy, hypogonadism, macrocytic anaemia
- Autoimmune diseases – vitiligo, skin rash, vasculitis
- Wilson's disease – Kayser–Fleisher rings, cirrhosis, tremor, dysarthria and dementia
- Polycystic kidney disease – bilateral mass in the flanks or previous nephrectomy (p. 41)
- Steatohepatitis

Symptoms

- Abdominal discomfort and swelling
- Related to underlying cause

Initial investigations

- FBC, ESR
- U+E, LFTs, including gamma-glutamyltransferase (γ-GT)
- Prothrombin time (PT), activated partial thromboplastin time (APTT) and thrombin time (TT)
- Abdominal ultrasound
- CXR

Subsequent investigations

- Cirrhosis (see p. 52)
- ECG and echocardiography
- Malignant disease – CT/MRI scanning, α-fetoprotein (hepatocellular cancer), biopsy
- Hepatitis serology

Management

- Depends on the cause

Points of interest

- Hepatitis:
  - Hep. A – transient disease which does not cause chronic disease but may very rarely cause fulminant hepatic failure and death.
  - Hep. B – 10% of cases may progress to chronic carrier states or chronic hepatitis. There is an increased risk of hepatocellular carcinoma with chronic hepatitis, and regular ultrasounds are required.
  - Hep. C – rarely causes acute hepatitis, but commonly results in cirrhosis.
  - Hep. D – associated only with Hep. B, causing more severe disease.
  - Hep. E – water-borne, causing epidemics; can be fatal to the mother in pregnancy.

6. CIRRHOSIS

Points in the examination

- Hands and skin – finger clubbing, leuconychia, spider naevi, palmar erythema, Dupuytren's contracture, jaundice, hepatic flap, scratch marks, pigmentation
- Eyes and face – pallor, jaundice, xanthelasma, parotid enlargement, peripheral cyanosis
- Abdomen – ascites, gynaecomastia, testicular atrophy, splenomegaly, hepatomegaly
- Legs – hair loss and oedema

Complications

- Portal hypertension – dilatation of abdominal veins, splenomegaly and ascites; will result in anaemia associated with gastrointestinal (GI) bleeding
- Encephalopathy – coarse flapping tremor, hepatic fetor, asterixis (inability to draw a 5-pointed star) and brisk reflexes
- Ascites (see p. 53)

Aetiology

Alcohol

- Parotid enlargement
- Multiple fractures
- Biopsy shows fatty infiltration in the early stages and Mallory's hyaline changes which occur with micronodular cirrhosis.

Viral hepatitis (usually biopsy + curettage (B+C))

- IV drugs, tattoos
- Associated with a macronodular cirrhosis

Autoimmune

- Occurs most commonly in women in their late 20s.
- Hepatomegaly and cirrhosis are characteristic.
- Other autoimmune conditions, e.g. fibrosing alveolitis.
- Antinuclear and anti-smooth-muscle antibodies are positive.

Primary biliary cirrhosis

- Occurs in middle-aged women, hepatomegaly and cirrhosis, associated with other autoimmune diseases.
- IgM, antimitochondrial and antinuclear antibodies are positive.

Haemochromatosis

- Autosomal recessive
- Occurs predominantly in 40–60-year-old men
- Liver biopsy reveals excess iron deposits
- Bronzed skin, diabetes mellitus, cirrhosis, hepatomegaly, arthritis, pituitary disease, impotence and gonadal atrophy

Wilson's disease

- Autosomal recessive – excess copper in the liver and basal ganglia
- Cirrhosis, Kayser–Fleisher rings, hepatomegaly, tremor, dysarthria and dementia
- Low serum copper, high 24-h urine copper
- Treatment is with penicillamine, which is often associated with deterioration in neurological function; relatives should be screened.

α_1-Antitrypsin deficiency

- Autosomal dominant
- Cirrhosis, hepatomegaly, and lung emphysema

Symptoms

- Fatigue and weight loss
- Icterus ± dark urine
- Pruritus
- Haematemesis and melaena – oesophageal varices
- Confusion associated with encephalopathy

Initial investigations

- U+E, LFT, γ-GT, FBC, glucose
- Prothrombin time, ± APTT, TT
- Liver ultrasound
- Liver biopsy

Subsequent specific investigations

- ANA, dsDNA, anti-smooth-muscle and mitochondrial antibodies
- 24-h urinary copper and serum caeruloplasmin
- Serum ferritin
- Viral hepatitis serology (hep. B and hep. C)
- α_1-Antitrypsin levels
- Immunoglobulins (raised IgM in PBC (primary biliary cirrhosis))
- EEG for encephalopathy

Management

- Pruritis – cholestyramine.
- Nutritional support – low-protein diet, low sodium.
- Alcohol abuse – abstinence, Antabuse, counselling.
- PBC – cholestyramine, ursodeoxycholic acid, liver transplant.
- Hepatitis B and C – α-interferon and antiretroviral therapy for active disease.
- Autoimmune disease – steroids, azathioprine.
- Haemochromatosis – venesection.
- Liver transplantation is the optimal treatment in endstage disease.
- Portal hypertension – β-blockade, recurrent sclerotherapy or transjugular intrahepatic portosystemic stent (TIPS).
- Encephalopathy – there are four grades of encephalopathy:
  - A simple tremor or flap
  - Confused but able to talk in sentences
  - Confused and unable to talk in sentences
  - Coma.
- In cirrhosis, encephalopathy is usually precipitated by an alcohol binge, infection, GI bleed, protein excess or constipation.
- Other causes of confusion in these patients include subdural haemorrhage, Wernicke's encephalopathy or alcohol withdrawal. Management requires specialist input but is essentially supportive: avoidance and treatment of the precipitant, low-protein diet, plus lactulose and neomycin.

7. ASCITES

Points in the examination

- Abdominal distension
- Everted umbilicus
- Shifting dullness

Aetiology

Transudate

- Cirrhosis – signs of chronic liver disease (including visible veins on the abdomen) ± hepatomegaly and encephalopathy
- Cardiac failure – oedema, raised JVP, shortness of breath, third heart sound
- Constrictive pericarditis – elevated JVP with rapid x and y descent, impalpable apex, quiet or normal heart sounds, loud S_3 'pericardial knock'
- Nephrotic syndrome – generalised oedema, proteinuria

Exudates

- Malignant disease – cachexia, lymphadenopathy, associated surgery, hepatomegaly
- Infection – pyrexia, tenderness:
  - Spontaneous bacterial peritonitis
  - Tuberculosis
- Hypothyroidism (see p. 408)

Differential diagnosis

- Obesity
- Pregnancy
- Constipation

Symptoms

- Cachexia/anorexia
- Weight gain
- Abdominal distension
- Shortness of breath
- Related to the cause

Initial investigations

- Ascitic tap (diagnostic paracentesis) – protein, cytology, MC+S (microscopy, culture and sensitivity), amylase
- LFT
- U+E
- Glucose
- FBC
- Blood culture
- Prothrombin time

Specific investigations

- Liver ultrasound
- CXR
- ECG and echo
- Urinary 24-h protein content
- Thyroid function tests

Management

- Paracentesis
- Low-salt diet and fluid restriction
- Diuretics – spironolactone, amiloride
- Treat underlying cause
- TIPS – joins the portal vein to the hepatic vein. Used predominantly in cirrhotic disease, but it can aggravate encephalopathy. However, it does seem to result in a survival advantage over paracentesis alone.

Points of interest

- Hepatocellular carcinoma:
  - 5% of patients with cirrhosis develop hepatocellular carcinoma
  - Associated with a rising α-fetoprotein (AFP) level and a sudden deterioration in liver function
  - A minority of patients can be treated with surgical resection
  - Other treatment options include chemoembolisation or even hepatic transplantation
  - The disease metastasises to lung and bone
  - There is no well-established role for chemotherapy or radiotherapy.
- Mechanism of ascites in cirrhosis:
  - Splanchnic vasoconstriction:
    - (i) decreased renal blood flow, causing (ii) secondary hyperaldosteronism, and thus (iii) salt and water retention, leading to (iv) reduced colloid osmotic pressure
    - the exact mechanism is unknown, but a combination of the above are all implicated.

STATION 2

The History-taking Examination

The History-taking Examination

GENERIC HISTORY-TAKING SKILLS

Introduction

History-taking is a special form of communication in which both parties are studying each other. It is one of the cornerstones of a doctor's skills. Although many candidates may already feel skilled in this discipline, the history-taking station in PACES is one that is commonly failed. This is usually due to poor technique, organisation or not covering all areas. Whilst taking a history is relatively straightforward in the safety of your own casualty or outpatients department, in the PACES exam all the rules change, perhaps comparable to playing Manchester United away, with a one-sided referee!

The aims of the history-taking station are to assess the candidate's ability to gather and assimilate information from the patient, and then to discuss the case with a 'colleague'. The following skills are considered:
- To elicit the presenting complaint in a logical and systematic way and to include a systems' review
- To enquire about past medical history, family, smoking, alcohol, treatment history
- To have the ability to follow leads about relevant psychosocial factors
- To demonstrate the appropriate use of verbal and non-verbal (posture, eye-contact, etc.) signs, responsiveness, to use a good balance of open and closed questions and to conduct the proceedings at an appropriate pace.

Key features of the station

- Written instructions for the case, usually in the form of a letter from the patient's GP, are given to the candidate to read in the 5-minute interval before the station.
- 14 minutes are allowed for the history-taking, 1 minute to collect one's thoughts and then 5 minutes for discussion – during which the patient is asked to leave the room.

- The examiners are present throughout and observe the history-taking. Although they have guidelines as to the key areas on which they base their overall mark, one is not marked on the specific points.
- There is potentially a vast amount of information to be gathered in a history. Not all of it can, or needs to be, collected in each case. The skill of taking a history is extracting the useful information from the patient to address his/her problems.

General approach

- Read the instructions carefully in the 5-minute interval before the station. Based on the symptoms given, consider the possible differential diagnoses to enquire about. If a medical condition is stated, consider its medical and social implications, associations with other conditions, complications and treatment.
- It is essential to try to put the patient at ease and encourage him/her to talk freely.
- Common courtesy goes a long way towards this. Greet the patient, by name if possible, and tell them who you are. The value of the patient's history and their confidence in you as a physician depends upon the rapport that is created.
- When the patient is telling the story, watch their gestures and the non-verbal clues, as it is as important to listen to what is not said, as to what is said, and how it is said. Make it clear from your posture, gestures and expression that the patient has your undivided attention. Don't sit there staring at the examiners, or out of the window, or spend the whole time furiously writing notes.
- Remember to use a mixture of open and closed questions. Start the consultation with a series of open questions, i.e. ones that do not suggest a particular answer, e.g. 'Why have you come to see me today?' or 'Tell me what is wrong from your point of view'. Move towards more closed questions as you progress in the history, e.g. 'Any trouble with your waterworks?' You may eventually need to use closed questions where the answer is suggested, e.g. 'When you wake at night are you thirsty?'

Taking a history in PACES

By convention, a medical history is recorded under the following headings:
1. Age, marital status, occupation/social circumstances
2. Presenting complaints
3. History of presenting complaints

4. Past medical history, including ongoing conditions
5. Treatment history
6. Social and occupational history
7. Family history
8. Review of systems, including menstrual history in women

It is essential that each of the separate headings comprising the full history is covered carefully in turn. It is the failure to do so and the omission of whole sections, such as family or drug history, that are common reasons for failing this station.

Presenting complaints

Although there is no one technique of history-taking that is applicable to each situation, or patient, having introduced oneself and established the patient's identity, age, occupation, and marital status and made them feel at ease, it is wise to open the consultation with a general open question such as: 'I have a letter from your GP, but first I would like you to tell me, in your words, what I can do for you (or what is the trouble)?' The patient should feel free to talk, and say what he wants from the consultation. This may take no more than a couple of minutes. It is essential to know in the patient's own words what the complaint is. So, the patient presents with 'my breathing', not dyspnoea.

For each symptom, establish the duration, severity, exacerbating and relieving factors, and the associated symptoms. If the presenting complaint is pain, you must additionally determine its site, character, radiation and timing.

Within the various systems, there are certain key questions that must be asked. Those detailed in the next section are a guide to these questions: the candidate should not routinely plough through all of these in turn, but instead will be assessed on their ability to draw out the relevant details of the complaint.

Remember that during history-taking the patient will not try and hide information from you. It is not a game of charades. If there are multiple presenting complaints, they should all be dealt with in sequence. For each one, make sure you ask:
- Have you seen other doctors for this problem?
- Have they told you what is wrong?
- What investigations have they done?
- Have they given you treatment in the past?

Ensure you have asked about the complications of any disease and, importantly, the social implications for each of the problems.

Past medical history

Enquire about previous surgery (reactions to anaesthetics if appropriate) and major illnesses. It is useful to specifically consider diabetes mellitus, hypertension, asthma, ischaemic heart disease, strokes, bronchitis/emphysema, tuberculosis, rheumatic fever, epilepsy, jaundice/liver disease and kidney disease.

Are there any other ongoing medical complaints for which they are receiving treatment, by whom and where? It is essential to ensure the follow-up of other conditions.

Treatment history

Include all details about ongoing and previous medical treatment and any matters arising from them. It is not just a list of current medications and their doses. Enquire about the side-effects of medications and any monitoring. Are they taking any over-the–counter medicines (e.g. aspirin, laxatives (including liquid paraffin))? Do they take anything else, including topical ointments, sprays or inhalers? Do they take any illicit drugs and, if so, what for – recreation or symptom relief, e.g. cannabis for pain in multiple sclerosis? Do they take herbal or homeopathic remedies, extracts or potions?

Social and occupational history

The social history is often the crux of the story. It is essential to remember that a patient is far more concerned with how their condition will affect their lifestyle or interfere with their activities of daily living (e.g. washing, dressing, feeding, shopping, etc.) and occupation than with the precise aetiology, as in: psoriatic or rheumatoid arthritis; congestive cardiac failure (CCF) secondary to ischaemic heart disease or cardiomyopathy; dyspnoea secondary to COPD or pulmonary fibrosis.

- Marital status – if single, do they have a partner? Is the spouse or partner well? Other family members, where they live, and if they visit. Does anyone else, e.g. a friend, neighbour, priest or doctor 'look in' or help with the shopping?
- What sort of place do they live in? If a flat, on which floor? Number of flights of stairs? Lifts, etc. Where is the toilet?

- What social and/or nursing services they have at home and how often:
  - Home help
  - Meals-on-wheels
  - District nurse
  - Twilight nursing.
- Determine how they manage with all activities of daily living (washing, dressing, eating, etc.). The list of potential avenues is endless, but the key thing is to get a feel for the patient's life, and for them to recognise that you are interested in how they cope with things.
- Find out the patient's occupation in detail and, if necessary, their full employment history from school. If chemicals are used, do they know their names? The following occupations and conditions are worthy of note for their associations or social implications:
  - Publicans and cirrhosis
  - Heavy-goods vehicle or public-service vehicle drivers and seizures
  - Machinery operators and the use of antihistamines or tranquillisers.
- Ask about smoking:
  - What do they smoke and how much? When did they start and how much have they smoked in the past? The above information will lead to numbers of pack-years:
    - 20 cigarettes a day for 10 years is 10 pack-years
    - 10 cigarettes a day for 10 years is 5 pack-years
    - 40 cigarettes a day for 10 years is 20 pack-years.
- Ask about alcohol consumption:
  - How much do they drink on average per week? Record in units/week
  - Go through a day's drinking, leaving nothing out. One unit is the equivalent of a glass of wine or half a pint of beer.

Family history

Enquire about any illnesses that run in the family. Ask about the age, health or cause of death of parents, siblings or children, if known. Questions about specific diseases related to the presenting complaint may be necessary, e.g. diabetes mellitus, ischaemic heart disease, breast cancer or hypertension. If a familial condition is postulated it may be necessary to go into greater detail about other more distant relatives or, in the limited time of the PACES, earmark it for later consideration on the problem list.

Review of systems

A common problem in PACES is history-taking of the presenting complaint in such detail that little time is left for the other components of the history. A good way of starting this section is to ask: 'Is there anything in your medical health that we have missed out or not talked about?'

A thorough history must include a review of the systems; the questions of importance can be extracted from the systems in the next section. One is essentially screening, and therefore the questions must probe for conditions of a high enough frequency or of sufficient seriousness that missing them would be detrimental. This information can either be gathered after the history of the presenting complaint or left to the end of the history. Although not the usual format, one benefit of taking it earlier is that unexpected important symptoms will not be raised late in the 14 minutes of time available.

Concluding

- Try to have a moment to recap the details to the patient, thereby checking the details and jogging their memory for anything that may have been missed.
- Ask if there are any outstanding issues.
- Thank the patient by name.
- Now that you have gathered all the relevant information, it is vital that you organise the history in the remaining minute so as to present it in an ordered manner. Generate a problem list for each 'complaint', including the differential diagnosis, relevant investigations you would wish to perform (simple, non-invasive first) and strategies/management plans to solve the problem(s). The examiners' questions will revolve around these points.
- If the history was not completed during the consultation do not panic: all one can do is take a structured history in a polite and competent manner, and endeavour to use the time effectively.

To summarise

- Read the information carefully.
- Initially discuss the social background of the patient.
- Ask open questions about the presenting complaint.
- Ask open questions about other medical and social problems.
- Go through the history systematically.
- Ensure a detailed social history.
- Construct a problem list.

- Anticipate the examiners' questions.
- Consider further investigations and management.

Following this systematic, well-organised process for the history-taking station will ensure that both the referee and crowd will be on your side throughout the match!

QUESTIONS BY SYSTEMS

Cardiovascular system

Chest pain

- Angina:
  - Exertional, dull, central
  - Stable, unstable
  - Radiates to the neck, jaw or arm
  - Relieved by rest, oxygen or glyceryl trinitrate (GTN)
  - Exacerbated by cold weather, emotion and meals
- Pericardial:
  - Stabbing, retrosternal
  - Longer-lasting than angina
  - Related to posture and ventilation
- Non-cardiac:
  - Well-localised – pleuritic or musculoskeletal?
  - Dull, retrosternal but non-exertional – oesophageal or mediastinal?

Dyspnoea

- Unusual feeling of breathlessness on effort or at rest. If severe may lead to orthopnoea and paroxysmal nocturnal dyspnoea. Graded by the New York Heart Association (NYHA), grades 1–4:
  1. Normal activity unlimited
  2. Comfortable at rest but moderate activity limited
  3. All activity limited
  4. Unable to do anything without symptoms; may have symptoms at rest
- With acute pulmonary oedema, a pink frothy haemoptysis may occur.

Syncope

- Many causes (q.v. loss of consciousness in neurology)
- Cardiac – no aura, transient loss of consciousness (if cardiac syncope causes prolonged loss of consciousness the patient usually dies), pale during the attack, flushes during a rapid recovery (May be incontinent of urine, but incontinence of stools is highly suspicious of epilepsy)

Oedema

- Dependent and worsens throughout the day

Palpitations

- Rapid or gradual onset and offset?
- Dizziness or loss of consciousness
- Anxiety, sweats or flushing?

Respiratory system

Cough

- Productive:
  - Night or day
  - Sputum or blood:
    - volume, consistency/colour
    - haemoptysis – fresh or altered

Breathlessness

- At rest or on exertion?
- Consistent or intermittent?
- Exercise tolerance, distance or time – what can they do? Activities of daily living limited?

Added noises

- Where in cycle, constant or intermittent?

Weight loss

- Duration, how much, associated loss of appetite, loose clothing?

Hoarseness

- Onset and duration

Pain

- Duration and character, relieving/exacerbating factors?

Abdominal system

Appetite

- Increased or decreased, and why? – pain, anorexia or depression

Weight

- Increased or decreased, and why?

Pain

- Lower or upper gastrointestinal?
- Site, radiation, severity, duration
- Localised or diffuse
- Pain-free periods and their duration
- Relation to food/stools; other aggravating or relieving factors
- Does it occur at night or wake from sleep?
- Is it actually pain or discomfort or bloating?

Vomiting

- Frequency, amount, relation to pain, relieves the pain or not
- Is it actually vomiting – constriction of the abdominal muscles against the diaphragm, or regurgitation – constriction of the stomach against the pylorus?
- Colour, blood, 'coffee grounds', sour and frothy or the previous day's food

Flatulence

- Up or down? Does it relieve symptoms?

Waterbrash

- Excessive salivation and regurgitation of clear, tasteless fluid

Heartburn

- Determine exactly what the patient means, relation to food, relieving factors; does it occur on lying down; is it associated with a bitter taste in the mouth?

Dysphagia

- Does it affect fluids? If so, this suggests a stricture; if not, is it achalasia or a neurological problem?
- Is swallowing difficult, or is there coughing? This may be bulbar palsy or pseudobulbar palsy.
- Is the dysphagia painful, constant or worsening? This suggests a malignant cause.
- Does the neck bulge on swallowing or is there gurgling? This may be a pharyngeal pouch.

Stools

- Change in habit
- Frequency – diarrhoea
- How many times and when?
- Related to meals or specific foods?
- Colour, formed, unformed, porridge-like, frothy, watery?
- Float, can they be flushed away?
- Do laxatives, beer or spicy foods bring it on?
- Codeine taken for diarrhoea at any time?
- Blood, slime or pus in the stool
- Alternating diarrhoea and constipation

Jaundice

- Jaundice in the skin or the eyes, now or in the past
- Change in colour of the urine, stools, or itch
- Other cases or a family history
- Tattoos, travel, operations, blood transfusions, recent ingestion of shellfish
- Medications – prescription, over-the-counter, herbal, illicit (especially intravenous), or anaesthetics
- Sexual preference, unprotected intercourse, partners

Mood

- Depression in the past or present (depression is a common association with pancreatic malignancy and irritable bowel syndrome)

Neurology

Headaches

- Sudden onset – subarachnoid haemorrhage, migraine, meningitis
- Insidious – raised intracranial pressure
- Circadian variation, worsens with coughing or straining – space-occupying lesion
- Precipitants, e.g. contraceptive pill and migraine or cortical venous thrombosis. Food, alcohol, intercourse
- Features of meningitis – neck stiffness, photo- and phonophobia
- Seizures, loss of consciousness
- What are their fears?
- Any head injury? Any litigation pending? Work situation

Blackouts

- Distinguishing the causes of loss of consciousness/funny turns is of paramount importance. Is it a seizure or cardiac syncope? Epilepsy can occur at any time, even lying down or at night. Often an aura. May become cyanosed during the attack, and may have abnormal movements. Often injury or the feeling of being battered and bruised. Both faecal and urinary incontinence may occur. Attacks can be prolonged, and recovery can be slow, with prolonged confusion or sleepiness. Amnesia is likely. May be residual paresis (Todd's paresis).
- If they are epileptiform, when did the first occur? Detailed description of first episode, often a witness is necessary. How long to the second seizure? What kind of epilepsy is it? Onset as generalised or focal? Induced, e.g. alcohol, flickering lights? During sleep? Birth/delivery history. Head injury/trauma. Earache/discharge.
- Differential diagnosis (q.v. syncope): syncope – vasovagal, Stokes–Adams; postural hypotension (consider autonomic neuropathy, drugs, venous insufficiency and steroid deficiency); carotid sinus hypersensitivity – on turning head or carotid sinus massage; vertebrobasilar ischaemia – with vertigo and brainstem signs; micturition and cough syncope; hypoglycaemia; raised intracranial pressure; hyperventilation; alcohol/drug use; factitious.

Weakness

- Paraparesis or hemiparesis. NB. cardiovascular risk factors.
- Handedness must be asked in all cases.
- Duration of onset, does it come and go?
- If paraparesis, any change in bladder or bowels?

Vertigo

- Deafness and/or tinnitus
- Nausea and vomiting
- Brainstem features
- Diplopia, bilateral visual obscurations, bilateral numbness or paraesthesia, bilateral facial weakness, limb weakness

Miscellaneous

- Speech – dysarthria (difficulty articulating), dysphasia (language difficulties)
- Swallowing, regurgitation, coughing
- Sleep, mood
- Travel, sexually transmitted diseases, exposure to poisons
- Family history

Musculoskeletal

- Arthritis, swelling, acute or chronic
- Which joints and when, with movement or at rest, palindromic?
- Morning stiffness – suggestive of active inflammation
- Pattern – first affected, symmetrical, monoarthropathy/polyarthropathy
- Small joints (proximal interphalangeal joints – rheumatoid arthritis or psoriatic arthritis; distal interphalangeal joints – osteoarthritis, gout or psoriasis)
- Large joints (osteoarthritis)
- Sacroiliitis. HLA B27. Psoriasis, inflammatory bowel disease, ankylosing spondylitis, SLE, dermatomyositis, scleroderma, erythema nodosum?
- Eyes – Sjögren's, conjunctivitis, uveitis
- Men – urethral discharge, women – vaginal discharge, suggesting Reiter's
- Gout
- Bone pain – does it occur during the day or at night?
- Family history
- Non-specific features of inflammation – fevers, malaise, weight loss, lethargy

Miscellaneous points

Sexual history

- Sexuality
- Number of partners
- Contraception/protection
- Previous STDs
- Previous investigations for STDs, inc. HIV test
- Previous treatment for STDs
- Treatment of partners

Haematological

- Lassitude, dyspnoea, palpitations, infections
- Blood loss – gums, epistaxis, bruises, rectal, melaena, menstrual. Spontaneous or out of proportion to the injury?
- Purpura or pigmentation
- Diet
- Glandular enlargement
- Particular attention to drug history, family history, occupational history

Urine

- Frequency – day or night, volume, thirst, decide on polyuria or frequency; prostatic problems or obstetric problems
- Urine volume altered, nocturia, incontinence, poor stream, colour, blood, turbid or frothy, if blood – where in the stream?
- Lumbar pain radiating to the groin, stranguary – 'the distressing desire to pass that which will not pass'
- Analgesic use
- Headache, vomiting, drowsiness, fits, diminished vision, dyspnoea
- Oedema (e.g. puffy face in the morning), dysuria, rheumatic fever, chorea, tonsillitis, purpura

Skin

- Where is the rash?:
  - Hands and feet – eczema, psoriasis, contact dermatitis
  - Finger webs – scabies, eczema, irritant dermatitis.
  - Face:
    - eczema and photosensitive rashes (worse in summer and sparing under chin and behind ears)
    - rosacea if across nose and around eyes (spares nasolabial folds)
    - lupus/sarcoid – ears/nose

- Mouth – pemphigus/lichen planus/
  Behçet's/Crohn's/herpes/*Candida*/Stevens–Johnson
  syndrome/Kaposi's sarcoma/amyloid/Addison's
- Flexor surfaces – eczema, drug rashes, acanthosis nigricans
- Extensor surfaces – psoriasis, but usually involves other areas,
  dermatitis herpetiformis, plus buttocks
- Legs – lichen planus (also wrists), varicose eczema, Graves'
  dermopathy, vasculitis.
- How long has the rash been present? Has it occurred before?
  Psoriasis/eczema/urticaria/connective tissue disease are usually of
  long standing. A rash of rapid onset is much more likely to have a
  specific cause, e.g. drug reaction, viral exanthema.
- Does the rash itch (e.g. eczema, urticaria, scabies, lichen planus,
  insect bites, fungal, bullous pemphigoid, cellulitis)?
- Does the rash blister (e.g. bullous pemphigoid, eczema, herpes,
  drugs, cellulitis, staphylococcal (impetigo), scalded skin)? Blisters in
  bullous pemphigoid are usually symmetrically distributed on the
  thighs and abdomen. They do not usually burst, unlike pemphigus.
- Is the rash painful (e.g. herpes, pustular/unstable psoriasis, early
  toxic epidermal necrolysis (TEN), lupus, vascular ulceration,
  erythema multiforme)? Painful rashes are not common – always think
  herpesvirus infection, esp. shingles.
- Does the rash improve (e.g. eczema, psoriasis), or worsen in the sun
  (e.g. lupus, dermatomyositis, drug-induced photosensitivity, rosacea,
  porphyria)?
- Ulcers are common. The causes can often be distinguished from the
  history.
    - Venous insufficiency (most common – previous surgery/DVT/
      varicose veins/eczema).
    - Arterial insufficiency (usually associated with other symptoms/
      signs of vascular disease).
    - Neuropathic – classically painless, punched out, plantar
      (e.g. diabetes).
    - Malignant – basal-cell carcinoma (BCC).
    - Genital – Behçets, syphilis ('Hunterian chancre').
- Past medical history:
    - Atopy – asthma/eczema/hay fever as child or now; long-term sun
      exposure – skin cancers
    - Systemic disease – many are associated with skin manifestations,
      e.g. Crohn's, SLE, sarcoid
    - Malignancy – associated with paraneoplastic skin manifestations,
      e.g. dermatomyositis
    - Social/occupational history – habits, diet, clothing, washing and
      occupation. Hobbies, exposure to animals, insects or plants?

- Drugs – does the rash coincide with starting or changing medication? Precipitants (e.g. β-blockers and lithium can exacerbate psoriasis)? Previous treatments – both prescribed and self-administered. If worsening with topical steroids – consider infection.
- Family history – psoriasis/atopy; infections, e.g. scabies, lice.

Endocrinology

- Malaise – thyrotoxicosis, insulin-dependent diabetes, adrenal failure
- Weight gain – hypothyroidism, Cushing's syndrome, growth-hormone deficiency
- Menstrual irregularity – prolactinoma, thyroid dysfunction, polycystic ovarian dysfunction, hypopituitarism, anorexia, pregnancy
- Impotence and loss of libido must be distinguished – diabetes mellitus, prolactinoma, stress (psychosocial), drugs and alcohol, primary and secondary hypogonadism
- Proximal muscle wasting or weakness – thyrotoxicosis, Cushing's, acromegaly
- Sleep disturbance/hypersomnolence – hypothyroidism, growth-hormone deficiency or insomnia, Cushing's, thyrotoxicosis
- Pigmentation – buccal, skin creases or scars suggesting Addison's disease or adrenocorticotrophic hormone (ACTH) excess; haemochromatosis – general slate-grey appearance
- Hirsutism, in association with oligomenorrhoea, infertility, obesity – polycystic ovarian syndrome, also Cushing's disease. Virilisation can rarely be caused by adrenal or ovarian androgen-secreting tumours, and congenital adrenal hyperplasia
- Pituitary disease:
  - Mass effects – headache or visual disturbance
  - Systemic effects of either pituitary hyper- or hypofunction, diabetes insipidus or hypothalamic dysfunction (failure to regulate temperature, thirst, satiety, sleep and memory)
  - Acromegaly (distal largeness – see p. 410)
  - Prolactinoma – galactorrhoea, oligo/amenorrhoea, decreased libido and infertility
  - Cushing's disease (see Cushing's syndrome – p. 413)
  - ACTH deficiency – fatigue, depression, postural dizziness (unusual as mineralocorticoid function preserved)
  - Growth hormone deficiency – fatigue, visceral/centripetal weight gain, muscle weakness, feeling of decreased well-being
  - Thyroid-stimulating hormone (TSH) deficiency – q.v. hypothyroidism

- Luteinising hormone(LH)/follicle-stimulating hormone (FSH) deficiency – impotence, infertility and amenorrhoea
  - Diabetes insipidus – polyuria, nocturia and thirst
- Primary hypothyroidism – insidious onset, weight gain, constipation, cold intolerance, menorrhagia, hoarse voice, lethargy, depression, forgetfulness and, rarely, dementia
- Hyperthyroidism – weight loss in the face of increased appetite, frequent stools, oligomenorrhoea, tremor, palpitations, irritability, emotional lability, heat intolerance, sweating, itch, proximal myopathy
- Hypercalcaemia – abdominal pain, nausea, vomiting, constipation, polyuria, anorexia, weight loss, polydipsia, fatigue, weakness, hypertension, confusion, cardiac arrest, stones, renal failure, corneal calcification
- Hypertension – always consider secondary causes:
  - Drugs, renovascular, renal parenchymal or endocrine causes. Mineralocorticoid excess, i.e. primary aldosteronism, is common, 5–10% in some series
  - Phaeochromocytoma is a rare cause of hypertension with palpitations, headache, sweating on a cool skin, with feelings of anxiety and impending doom
  - Pointers for secondary hypertension should be young age of onset, difficult control using multiple agents, or family history of hypertension
  - Biochemically – an alkalosis with or without hypokalaemia
- Carcinoid syndrome – vague abdominal symptoms, often diarrhoea and flushing, breathlessness, murmurs (classically right-sided)

Diabetes mellitus

- When and where diagnosed?
- Who is following up, and when seen last?
- Home blood or urine monitoring, results?
- Hypoglycaemia? Aware? Frequency? Nocturnal?
- High sugars? Admissions, ketosis, coma, HONK?
- Current medications – how are they taken, side-effects?
- Lifestyle, diet and exercise?
- Diabetes nurse follow-up, dietician, chiropodist?
- Osmotic symptoms?
- Complications:
  - Macrovascular:
    - coronary heart disease
    - cerebrovascular disease
    - peripheral vascular disease

- Microvascular:
  - retinopathy, maculopathy
  - nephropathy
  - neuropathy ± postural hypotension
- Feet
- Neuropathic ulcers
- Charcot's joints
- Impotence
- Smoking, lipids
- Hypertensive?
- Job and driving

HIV/AIDS

History of present complaint

- Date, location and mode of transmission (intravenous drug user (IVDU), homosexual, heterosexual)
- Date of previous negative test, date of positive test
- Initial and subsequent CD4 counts/viral load
- Subsequent opportunistic infections and cancers
- Treatments received for these infections
- Current prophylaxis against infections (PCP prophylaxis if CD4 <200; MAC prophylaxis if CD4 <50)
- Hepatitis B+C status
- AIDS-defining diagnoses

Treatment – highly active antiretroviral therapy (HAART)

- Drug combinations – past and present
- Side-effects and allergies
- Drug resistance

Social history

- Sexual history – including partners and safe sex. Ask about HIV status of partners.
- Does their partner know they are HIV-positive?
- Are any other members of the family HIV-positive (children)?
- Do family, friends and work know the diagnosis?
- Are they in touch with support groups?
- What pets are at home?

Drug history

- HAART
- Prophylaxis against opportunistic infections
- Recreational drugs
- Alcohol

2

History-taking Scenarios

1. Abnormal liver function tests
2. Epigastric pain
3. Chronic cough
4. Chest pain
5. Breathlessness
6. Blackout
7. Diarrhoea
8. Hypertension
9. Tuberculosis
10. Loss of consciousness
11. Pain
12. Crohn's disease
13. Haemoptysis
14. HIV-related headache
15. Asthma
16. Atrial fibrillation
17. Weak legs
18. Headache – 1
19. Headache – 2
20. Small-joint arthropathy
21. Malabsorption
22. Nephrotic syndrome

1. ABNORMAL LIVER FUNCTION TESTS

A 43-year-old businesswoman has been referred by the casualty officer with abnormal LFTs. The lady was alert and orientated but did have some right upper quadrant tenderness.

Please take a history.

Diagnoses to consider

- Alcoholic liver disease
- Viral hepatitis
- Primary biliary cirrhosis/autoimmune hepatitis
- Gilbert's syndrome
- Drugs
- Obstructive causes – gallstones, pancreatic cancer, liver metastasis
- Haemochromatosis

Points in the history

History of present complaint (HPC)

- Constitutional symptoms or episodes of jaundice (especially with fasting)
- Travel abroad, unusual foods (shellfish associated with Hepatitis A), blood transfusions and IV drugs (Hep. B and C), sexual history (Hep. B, C and D)
- Alcohol intake (see later)
- Change in colour of stools and urine suggesting an obstructive cause
- Weight loss, new lumps, changes in bowel habit, unusual blood discharge, previous smear/mammogram investigations – associated with malignancy
- Last menstrual period (LMP) and possibility of pregnancy (Hep. E)
- Arthralgia and skin pigmentation – haemochromatosis

Past medical history (PMH)

- Liver disease
- Abdominal surgery
- Abdominal pain or gallstones
- Autoimmune diseases
- Diarrhoea – associated with Crohn's, ulcerative colitis
- Previous malignancy

Drugs

- IV drugs
- Herbal remedies
- Regular prescriptions
- Over-the-counter medications, etc.

Family history

- Liver disease
- Malignancies
- Autoimmune disease
- Gilbert's syndrome

Sexual history

- Including contraception and HIV risk

Social history

- Ask about smoking and alcohol.

Alcohol history

Individuals can be sensitive about their alcohol intake. Doctors should not appear judgemental. If the doctor appears impartial, the patient is more likely to be honest – e.g. 'Lots of people drink more than the recommended amount without it affecting their day-to-day life; do you drink more than is recommended?' (Current guidelines suggest a maximum weekly intake of 14 units for women and 21 units for men.)

- How much and what type (spirits, wine, beer)?
- If she is drinking much more than the recommended limit ask the following:
  - Where, when and with whom?
  - How does it affect your:
    - domestic life – relationship, friends, home and children
    - work life – recent redundancies, drinking at work
    - financial situation – jobs, mortgages, etc.?
- Other questions:
  - Precipitating factors – relationship, work?
  - Binge drinking?
  - Has she sought help before?
  - Violence or trouble with the police?

- Specific questions:
  - Have you tried to reduce the amount you drink?
  - Do you get angry if people tell you that you drink too much?
  - Do you feel guilty about how much you drink?
  - Do you ever drink in the mornings?
  - These four questions are well-established discriminatory questions which point towards alcoholism. It is known as the CAGE questionnaire:
    - C – cut down
    - A – angry
    - G – guilty
    - E – early morning drinking

Review of systems

Investigations

- LFTs, γ-GT, prothrombin time
- FBC – macrocytes, thrombocytopenia
- Viral hepatitis serology
- Autoimmune profile – ANA, antimitochondrial and smooth-muscle antibodies, liver–kidney microsomal (antibody)-1 (LKM1)
- Serum electrophoresis – IgM in PBC, hypergammaglobulinaemia in autoimmune hepatitis
- Liver ultrasound – fatty change, dilated biliary tree or metastatic disease

Management

- If alcohol-related – abstention should be encouraged. Offer counselling and group sessions. Alcoholics Anonymous, etc.
- Primary biliary cirrhosis is treated with ursodeoxycholic acid, but liver transplantation is usually required at some stage.
- Autoimmune liver disease may respond to steroids and other immunosuppressants.
- Haemochromatosis is treated with venesection and desferrioxamine.
- Otherwise treat the cause.

Points of interest

- Gilbert's syndrome is an autosomal dominant disease affecting 5% of the population. It usually presents before the age of 25 and is caused by a defect in the enzyme UDP-glucuronyltransferase. Jaundice is precipitated by stress, fasting and illness. The bilirubin is unconjugated.
  - Investigate with a prolonged fast, resulting in a raised unconjugated bilirubin, although it is rarely necessary.

2. EPIGASTRIC PAIN

A GP letter to gastroenterology outpatients:

This pleasant 55-year-old male car salesman has recently been made redundant. He has been suffering from epigastric pain for the last few months that has not responded to antacids. Please advise.

Diagnoses to consider

- Oesophageal reflux
- Peptic ulcer
- Upper GI cancer
- Depression
- Cardiac pain
- Pancreatitis
- Gallstones

Approach to the patient

Candidates should be aware that although this gentleman had a specific medical complaint, there is also an important social issue (losing his job). Questions should be asked about this issue early on in the consultation, as it may have precipitated his medical condition.

Points in the history

HPC

- Duration, site, radiation, alleviating factors, previous episodes, nausea and vomiting
- Previous GI investigations, e.g. endoscopy
- Weight loss – a good marker of pathology
- Haematemesis – almost always needs further investigation
- Melaena or change in bowel habit
- Be clear as to the timing of the symptoms and the redundancy. One may have precipitated the other
- Oesophageal reflux:
  - Retrosternal pain radiating to the arms, made worse with stooping or lying and often associated with nausea and regurgitation

- Gastric ulcer:
  - Epigastric pain radiating to the back, which is worse with food and tends to recur in bouts
- Duodenal ulcers:
  - Compared to gastric ulcers the patients are younger (in their 20s and 30s); more commonly associated with *Helicobacter pylori*; cause epigastric pain, radiating to the back that is often worse at night
- Gastric cancer:
  - Progressive constant epigastric pain made worse with food
- Evidence of cardiac type pain – i.e. with exercise

PMH

- Cardiac disease
- Depression

Drug history

- Precipitating drugs – non-steroidal anti-inflammatory drugs (NSAIDs) or alcohol
- Medication to alleviate symptoms

Family history

- Malignancy

Travel

- Increased incidence of *Helicobacter pylori* in the Third World

Social history

- How has the redundancy changed his life, how are things at home, how are things financially?
- Smoking and alcohol history

Review of systems

- Depression can cause a wide variety of medical symptoms, especially GI symptoms.
- Questions about this are sensitive, and often best left to the end of the consultation, by which time a good rapport has been established.
- It is important that the patient does not feel their symptoms are simply being attributed to mental illness.

Approach

'People often feel very low in their spirits after losing their job and find it difficult to bounce back, what about you?' If the answer is 'Yes' then more direct questions can be asked; otherwise one should tread much more carefully. Further questions may be best left to follow-up appointments.

The doctor should then move on to more discriminatory questions:
- Degree of depression – early morning waking, anything positive in the future?
- Duration of symptoms
- Poor concentration – which may have resulted in the redundancy
- Precipitating factors – relationships, redundancy, money, bereavement
- Coping strategies, e.g. alcohol
- Previous episodes
- How it affects his home life and personal relationships.

If patient is clearly profoundly depressed they should be assessed for suicide risk before leaving:
- 'Have you ever thought it's not worth going on?'
- If 'Yes': 'Have you considered taking your own life?'
- If 'Yes' look for intent: 'Have you made any plan to end your life or tried before?'

Investigations

- FBC, LFTs, calcium and glucose levels
- *Helicobacter* antibodies
- Endoscopy and CLO (CampyLObacter pylori – now reclassified as a helicobacter) test – leading to therapy for *Helicobacter pylori*
- ECG if cardiac cause is suspected
- If all the above are negative, consider liver ultrasound – gallstones and alcohol intake

Management

- Stop precipitating factors – smoking, stress, alcohol, NSAIDs.
- If the patient is depressed and not suicidal, professional counselling, a course of SSRIs (selective serotonin-reuptake inhibitors) and referral to the psychiatrists are appropriate.

3. CHRONIC COUGH

A 38-year-old man is referred to the respiratory clinic with a persistent, non-productive cough evident over the last 6 months.

Please take a history.

Diagnoses to consider

- Asthma
- Postnasal drip
- Postviral infection
- Oesophageal reflux/gastritis
- TB
- Lung cancer
- Sarcoid
- Drugs

Points in the history

HPC

- Duration of symptoms – patients often put up with a cough for many years
- Previous symptoms – asthma as a child (as it can recur in adulthood)
- Any other respiratory symptoms – e.g. haemoptysis (see p. 123)
- Postviral:
  - Flu-like symptoms, lymphadenopathy or preceding upper respiratory symptoms
- Asthma:
  - Timing of symptoms – worse at night, precipitated by exercise, emotion
  - Other respiratory symptoms – e.g. wheeze, shortness of breath, chest tightness
  - Allergies – e.g. house dust, cats
- Postnasal drip:
  - Symptoms of sputum running down the back of the throat
  - Unpleasant taste of sputum
  - Other ENT symptoms – blocked nose, etc.
- GI symptoms:
  - Heartburn, reflux, pain at night or with food, regurgitation

- Sarcoid:
  - Rashes, eye symptoms, glandular enlargement or shortness of breath
- Lung cancer/TB:
  - Weight loss, lethargy, haemoptysis, night sweats

PMH

- Childhood asthma – asthma often returns in the 4th decade
- Atopy – asthma which develops in middle-age is often not associated with atopy
- Nasal polyps
- Peptic ulcers
- ENT surgery or sinus problems

Drug history

- ACE inhibitors – common cause of chronic cough
- NSAIDs – can trigger asthma
- Inhalers

Family history

- Asthma/atopy
- Lung cancer

Social history

- Smoking history and exposure to passive smoking (social/ occupational exposure)
- Living conditions (overcrowding, damp housing)
- Exposure to pollution

Travel history

- TB endemic areas

Review of systems

Initial investigations

- FBC (eosinophilia), ESR
- CXR – to exclude lung cancer, sarcoid and TB
- Respiratory function tests (RFTs)
- U+E, LFTs, bone profile

- Allergen testing
- Serum ACE levels
- CT of sinuses – postnasal drip

Further investigations

- Peak-flow monitoring for morning dipping
- If the patient has GI symptoms a trial of proton-pump inhibitors and endoscopy may be required
- Bronchoscopy is not required unless CXR is abnormal or RFTs show a restrictive defect (will also require high-resolution CT scan)

Management

- If it is a postviral cough it may persist for several weeks. Reassurance is all that is required. May improve with inhaled steroids.
- If asthma is suspected a trial of a low-dose steroid inhaler is indicated.
- Postnasal drip requires ENT opinion.

Points of interest

Asthma often presents in middle-aged people as a chronic cough. Patients often had asthma as a child, which improved during their teens and then relapsed. However, it may present for the first time at this age. Adults presenting with asthma for the first time tend not to show atopy, unlike children.

Although chronic cough is a very common symptom, and is almost always due to a benign cause, it is essential to exclude significant pathology, such as lung cancer, even in this young gentleman. Very rarely, recurrent pulmonary emboli or even fibrosis may present with long-standing cough.

4. CHEST PAIN

You are the medical SHO on call and you have accepted the following referral from a GP:

Dear Colleague,
Please can you see this 49-year-old man who has recently been complaining of chest pains? His examination reveals a blood pressure of 140/96 mmHg.
Many thanks.

Please take a history from this patient.

Diagnoses to consider

- Ischaemic heart disease
  - Stable angina
  - Unstable angina
  - Myocardial infarction
- Pulmonary embolism
- Pericarditis
- Gastro-oesophageal pain
- Musculoskeletal pain

Points in the history

HPC

- Pain now?
- Consider the nature of the pain
- Angina:
  - Exertional, dull, central, radiating to the left arm or jaw, occurring at a predictable workload, with associated pallor, nausea, sweating or dyspnoea/orthopnoea, relieved by GTN, oxygen or rest
- Unstable angina:
  - Similar character, but occurring at rest or lower than expected workload, or increasing frequency or duration
- Myocardial infarction:
  - Vomiting, angor animi (feeling of impending doom), prolonged pain
- Pulmonary embolism (large proximal):
  - Similar pain associated with severe dyspnoea, relieved by lying flat, associated with immobility, malignancy, recent surgery, pregnancy, thrombophilia, prior DVT

- Pulmonary embolism (showers, small peripheral):
  - Pleuritic pain, associated with cough/haemoptysis, possibly dyspnoea, and risk factors above
- Pericarditis:
  - Pleuritic central pain, varying with posture, classically relieved by sitting forward, antecedent history of viral infection
- Gastro-oesophageal:
  - Cardiac 'type' pain but no relation to exertion, can be relieved by antacids or GTN
- Musculoskeletal:
  - Pleuritic-type pain with surface tenderness, antecedent trauma

PMH

- Previous cardiovascular disease, investigations and treatment
- Cerebrovascular or peripheral vascular disease
- Raised low-density lipoprotein (LDL), low high-density lipoprotein (HDL) cholesterol, hypertriglyceridaemia
- Diabetes mellitus
- Hypertension
- Risk factors for DVT
- Pericarditis: viral, pyogenic, tuberculous, malignant, uraemia, hypothyroid, associated with autoimmune disease, including acute rheumatic fever

Drug history

- Contraindications to aspirin, β-blockade, heparin, thrombolysis

Family history

- Peripheral vascular disease, smoking, thrombophilia, familial hypercholesterolaemia

Social history

- Smoking
- Implications for occupation and lifestyle
- Recent travel – DVT

Review of systems

Consider diagnoses that will exacerbate angina, e.g. anaemia, thyrotoxicosis, aortic stenosis, hypertrophic cardiomyopathy (HCM) and (especially in younger patients) cocaine abuse.

Initial investigations

- FBC – neutrophil leucocytosis and thrombocytosis in myocardial infarction (MI); lymphocytosis in viral or TB pericarditis
- ECG – normal at rest, or with ST depression in the offending territory during angina (compare if possible with previous ECGs); exclude MI. Flattened or biphasic T waves are non-specific but may offer a pointer. Features of pulmonary embolus – S1, Q3, T3, sinus tachycardia, right bundle-branch block (RBBB), (often normal); saddle-shape ST elevation of pericarditis
- Glucose
- Lipids
- ESR and CRP – may help diagnose and monitor pericarditis
- TSH and T_4
- CXR – normal or may show cardiomegaly from hypertension, or enlargement from valvular pathology
- Creatine kinase (CK) and later aspartate aminotransferase (AST) and lactate dehydrogenase (LDH) – as they define myocardial infarction with either a compatible history or ECG; however, each will be normal at the appropriate intervals
- Troponin I levels – unhelpful *per se* as it stratifies risk in individuals with ischaemic heart disease, rather than diagnosing myocardial infarction. However, in angina, a raised troponin level will identify a group of patients who may benefit from aggressive and early intervention

Further investigations (for ischaemic heart disease)

- Exercise test – useful with suspicious symptoms; exercise will induce ischaemia in stenoses of 70% or more. ST depression of 1 mm 80 ms after the J point is most characteristic of ischaemia, but symptoms and the workload at which they occur are important. The systolic blood presssure should rise by at least 20 mmHg; it may fail to rise in ischaemia and it is a grave sign if it falls. Development of ventricular ectopics may occur in disease
- Myocardial scintigraphy, e.g. thallium scan – if exercise testing unsuitable
- Angiography – cannot diagnose angina, but can show possible culprit lesions

Management

- Stable disease may be managed as an outpatient with modification of treatment and lifestyle changes.
- Unstable disease requires admission to a coronary care unit for oxygen, IV GTN, aspirin and low molecular-weight heparin. Aspirin is continued long-term.
- Nitrates are the first line of therapy for angina alongside opiates.
- β-blockers or calcium-channel blockers can also be added early. If symptoms are not controlled the patient should be stabilised and transferred for angiography, possibly with a view to intracoronary thrombolysis, angioplasty ± stenting or surgery. If there is a delay in these interventions then an intra-aortic balloon pump should be considered; these inflate during diastole causing an increase in the coronary perfusion pressure.
- Patients with diabetes require IV insulin.
- Hypercholesterolaemia total >5 mmol/l or LDL >3 mmol/l warrants treatment with a statin.
- In the medium- to long-term, modification of lifestyle is of paramount importance – smoking, exercise, diet.

Points of interest

- Antiplatelet agents – 300 mg of aspirin followed by 75 mg/day is undoubtedly beneficial in preventing secondary morbidity and mortality in all patients unless they have a definite contraindication to its use.
- Lipid lowering – statins have clearly demonstrated benefit not only in secondary prevention and primary prevention, but lowering cholesterol levels in asymptomatic individuals with a normal cholesterol has also been shown to be beneficial. *This is a rapidly changing area and candidates should be aware of the up-to-date recommendations in the UK.*
- Ramipril (and possibly other ACE inhibitors) reduces the incidence of stroke or a transient ischaemic attack (TIA) in patients at high risk of stroke, irrespective of their blood pressure.

5. BREATHLESSNESS

The following patient has been asked by his general practitioner to attend the hospital for emergency assessment:

Dear Doctor,
Please see this 60-year-old who has been complaining of nocturnal cough and breathlessness for the past 4 months. It has become increasingly debilitating over these last few days, such that he can no longer get about the house.

Please take a history from this patient.

Diagnoses to consider

- Congestive cardiac failure
- Asthma
- Chronic obstructive airways disease
- Malignancy
- Fibrosing alveolitis
- Recurrent pulmonary emboli

Points in the history

HPC

- Onset and duration of illness
- Dyspnoea
  - Functional ability now and at their best must be defined
  - Orthopnoea, paroxysmal nocturnal dyspnoea (PND), exercise tolerance
    - New York Heart Association (NYHA) grade
- Cough – dry or productive; associated wheeze
  - Sputum – frothy, purulent, haemoptysis
- Oedema
- Chest pain
- Weight loss
- Consider aetiology if CCF, especially:
  - IHD
  - Hypertension
  - Valvular disease
- DVT risk

PMH

Drug history

- Precipitants and treatments
- The common side-effects of treatment, e.g. anorexia and nausea (digoxin), gout, impotence, diabetes mellitus, hypokalaemic weakness (thiazides), postural hypotension (diuretics and all afterload reducing agents), dry cough and dysgeusia (ACE inhibitors), headache (nitrates)

Family history

Social history

- Smoking
- Alcohol – dilated cardiomyopathy
- Implications for occupation and lifestyle – activities of daily living (ADL), hobbies, sports, family life, sex life, ability to travel, etc.
- Occupational exposure – fibrosis

Review of systems

Reactive depression is very common in heart failure of any aetiology and must be specifically asked about.

Initial investigations

- FBC
- Urea, creatinine, electrolytes and bicarbonate
- Pulse oximetry ± arterial gases
- ECG – sinus tachycardia, atrial fibrillation, P. mitrale or pulmonale, left and/or right ventricular hypertrophy, old or current myocardial infarction or ischaemia, other arrhythmia precipitating the episode; heart failure is unlikely if ECG is normal
- CXR – left ventricular enlargement, if severe; also left atrial enlargement, pulmonary venous engorgement, pleural fluid, Kerley B lines and possible right ventricular and atrial enlargement
- Peak expiratory flow rate

Further investigations

- Echocardiography – essential to aid in a precise diagnosis, and will exclude a pericardial effusion

- Angiography – if there is a possibility that revascularisation may improve cardiac output
- Lung function tests, including transfer factor
- High-resolution CT – fibrosis
- V/Q scan or spiral CT – pulmonary emboli

Management (congestive cardiac failure)

- Depends on severity and duration.
- Acute and severe:
  - Oxygen, IV diuretics and nitrates, opiates, ± inotropes
  - If the picture is of cardiogenic shock then central venous pressure, intra-arterial and right heart pressure monitoring is appropriate in either an ITU or coronary-care unit (CCU) setting.
- Chronic heart failure:
  - Stop precipitants. Diuretics are the mainstay, alongside ACE inhibition, β-blockers (cautiously) and spironolactone. Control blood pressure, especially in diabetes (and glycaemia)
  - In clear-cut cases where the patient is relatively well, as is often the case in patients seen in clinic, management can be commenced as an outpatient
  - Give risk factor advice – smoking, physical activity, alcohol consumption and diet. Consider the potential benefit from: cardiac rehabilitation, palliative care services, long-term social support, transplantation
  - Influenza vaccination yearly and pneumococcal vaccine once.

Points of interest

- Pulmonary oedema does not automatically equate with left ventricular failure (LVF); it may occur in mitral stenosis with a perfectly normal ventricle. Similarly, LVF may occur in sepsis, myxoedema, hypoalbuminaemia, subarachnoid haemorrhage, gas inhalation or adult respiratory distress syndrome.
- It must not be overlooked that heart failure carries a poor prognosis. In the Framingham study the 5-year mortality for men was 62% and 42% for women with all degrees of heart failure. This information is often not clearly conveyed to the patient.
- Cardiogenic shock has a mortality of 80% and needs co-ordinated, rapid multidisciplinary input, on either a CCU or ITU, in the first 2 hours if the patient is to survive.

AETIOLOGICAL CONSIDERATIONS FOR HEART FAILURE

Ischaemic heart disease	
Hypertension	
Valvular disease	Rheumatic fever, infective endocarditis, Marfan's syndrome, lupus, seronegative arthritides (especially ankylosing spondylitis)
Cardiomyopathy	Dilated > hypertrophic
Infiltration	Amyloid, sarcoid, iron, rarely malignant
Infection	Viral myocarditis, rheumatic myocarditis, sepsis, infective endocarditis with myocarditis
Irradiation	For example, breast cancer, causing myocardial fibrosis
Drugs	For example, anthracyclines, 5-fluorouracil, Herceptin
Metabolic	Myxoedema, thyrotoxicosis, phaeochromocytoma, acromegaly, diabetes mellitus
Toxins	For example, alcohol
Pericardial effusion	Malignant, tuberculous, viral, renal failure, anticoagulation
Postpartum	
Nutritional	For example, beriberi, kwashiorkor, pellagra
Inherited	For example, Fabry's disease, muscular dystrophy, myotonic dystrophy, Friedreich's ataxia, storage diseases
Hypersensitivity	Anaphylactic shock
Cardiac transplant	Rejection
Persistent tachycardia	
Trauma	

6. BLACKOUT

Dear Colleague,
Please see this 79-year-old lady, who has had three falls. Apart from feeling
a little more tired than normal over the last few months she has been well.
I could find no injury and her examination was normal except for a pulse
of 40 beats per minute.

Please take a history.

Diagnoses to consider

- Heart block leading to bradycardia or tachycardia
- Sick-sinus syndrome
- Primary cerebral disease – space-occupying lesion, vascular disease, epilepsy
- Postural hypotension
- Critical aortic stenosis
- Carotid sinus hypersensitivity
- Hypothyroidism

Points in the history

HPC

- Distinguish between:
  - Falls and blackouts – a witness history may be helpful
  - Cardiac or neurological blackout (see pp. 66,69)
  - Syncope – secondary to arrhythmias or ventricular outflow obstruction
- Symptoms of ischaemic or valvular heart disease
- Postural hypotension – falls after standing up
- Cough syncope – in chronic bronchitis and emphysema ('laryngeal vertigo of Charcot')
- Micturition syncope – usually elderly men getting up from a warm bed to pass urine standing up; probably due to a combination of increased vagal tone and postural hypotension
- Carotid sinus hypersensitivity – syncope with tight collars, shaving (men), turning head
- Hypothyroidism – tired, weight gain, cold intolerance, dry skin and hair, impaired mentation
- Space-occupying lesion – headache, nausea, neurological symptoms
- Vestibular or cervical spine disease

PMH

- Cognitive impairment
- Parkinson's disease, visual impairment and sensory loss (impaired proprioception) may compound the problem
- Malignancy
- Endocrine or autoimmune disease

Drug history

- Sedatives, hypnotics
- Hypotensives or β-blockers

Social history

- Detailed social situation and premorbid condition are essential to determine subsequent management
- Consider loose flooring at home
- Alcohol
- Driving issues

Family history

- Can be important in arrhythmias, e.g. long QT syndrome

Review of systems

Initial investigations

- FBC, U+E, glucose, liver and bone profile
- ECG – heart block, sick-sinus syndrome, atrial fibrillation (AF), left ventricular hypertrophy (LVH)
- CXR – may reveal calcification in the cardiac silhouette, especially focused around the aortic valve; cardiomegaly and pulmonary plethora from chronic low output
- TSH, T_4
- 24-hour Holter monitoring – may be required if the ECG is non-diagnostic. Usually the indication for insertion of a permanent pacemaker is so compelling it may add little information. The nocturnal rate can be as low as 20 b.p.m. in complete heart block (CHB)

Further investigations

- CT brain with contrast – if primary cerebral disease suspected
- EEG
- Echocardiography

Management (heart block and sick-sinus syndrome)

- Insert a permanent pacemaker.
- Insertion is under local anaesthetic. They require regular checks. Depending on the system inserted, battery life may be up to 10 years.
- After a collapse, it is prudent to admit the patient for cardiac monitoring for the first 24 hours while permanent pacing is arranged. There may be no need to temporarily pace the myocardium at this stage.

Points of interest

- The most common aetiology of CHB is central bundle-branch fibrosis (Lenègre's disease), often with normal coronary arteries. Giddiness, transient amnesia, cognitive impairment and misdiagnosed epilepsy may all be due to atrioventricular (AV) block in the absence of syncope.
- In complete heart block, pacing should abolish symptoms and prolong life (1-year mortality: 35–50% unpaced; 5% paced). Therefore, once diagnosed, patients with CHB require a permanent pacemaker (PPM), even if asymptomatic, as the first symptom may be death.
- Mobitz II, symptomatic bi- and trifascicular block, and sick-sinus syndrome with documented spontaneous or drug-induced bradycardia warrant pacing.
- Permanent pacemakers cause little problem with day-to-day life, but MRI is contraindicated and diathermy must be used with caution.

7. DIARRHOEA

A letter has been sent from a local GP to the gastroenterology outpatients department:

This 39-year-old lady with a family history of colon cancer has suffered from intermittent diarrhoea over the last few months. Would you be kind enough to see her and advise on management?

Please take a history from this patient.

Diagnoses to consider

- Irritable bowel syndrome (IBS)
- Inflammatory bowel disease
- GI malignancy
- Infective diarrhoea
- Drugs – laxatives, alcohol
- Malabsorption
- Diverticular disease
- Thyrotoxicosis

Approach to the patient

- This lady is probably concerned about colonic cancer, and would like further investigations. Often patients with a family history of a disease are more sensitive to the symptoms.
- This lady should be reassured that while it is unlikely that these symptoms are related to cancer, they do require further investigation.

Points in the history

HPC

- How much, how often (>300 g/day for true diarrhoea)
- Symptoms at night and weight loss – suggests organic pathology
- Bloody or watery diarrhoea – colonic inflammation or cancer
- Pale and difficult to flush – steatorrhoea (malabsorption)
- Symptoms of thyroid disease – anxiety, palpitations, weight loss, tremor and heat intolerance
- Eye, skin or joint symptoms occur with inflammatory bowel disease

- A long history of intermittent and varying symptoms associated with abdominal pain are consistent with irritable bowel syndrome; it is often associated with stress, abdominal distension and psychological issues
- Onset – sudden, with a short history, suggests infection
- Recent travel also suggests infective causes

PMH

- Abdominal surgery
- Autoimmune diseases
- Depression (see before)

Drug history

- Laxatives, antibiotics and alcohol – common causes

Social history

- Stress and depression at home or work
- Smoking – protective of ulcerative colitis (UC), worsens Crohn's disease
- Alcohol

Family history

- A family tree should be drawn, with details of age of diagnosis of cancer, age of death and type of malignancy.
- First-degree relatives and younger affected individuals (<50 years) are more significant.

Review of systems

Investigations

- FBC, ESR, CRP LFT, U+E – signs of inflammation or chronic disease
- Stool volume and fat content over 24 hours
- Stool microscopy
- Sigmoidoscopy/colonoscopy and biopsy (in view of her family history)

Management (of irritable bowel syndrome)

- Diet – small frequent meals
- Exercise is often beneficial

- Psychological support
- Avoidance of life stresses
- Antispasmodics, antimotility and bulking agents can be helpful
- Many patients do not need regular follow-up

Points of interest

Screening for colonic cancer

Factors associated with an increased risk of colon cancer:
- First-degree relative with colon cancer
- First-degree relative with an adenoma when under the age of 60 years
- Personal history of breast or ovarian cancer
- Inflammatory bowel disease
- Acromegaly.

These account for 20% of cases of colon cancer.

Other rarer conditions have a particular increased risk:
- Familial adenomatous polyposis (FAP) – an autosomal dominant disease, resulting in the development of multiple colonic adenomatous polyps. Adenomas are thought to be an early step in the development of colon cancer.
- Hereditary non-polyposis colon cancer (HNPCC) is due to an abnormality in DNA-repair mechanisms resulting in a higher incidence of colon cancer, particularly right-sided cancers.

Together, they account for 6% of colon cancers.

All these patients should be screened at regular intervals with colonoscopy. The role of screening colonoscopy in the asymptomatic general population is controversial, although probably beneficial. Tumour markers such as carcinoembryonic antigen (CEA) do not have a role in colon cancer screening (unlike prostate-specific antigen (PSA) in prostate cancer).

Irritable bowel syndrome (IBS)

- 20% of adults have symptoms of IBS, which usually affects younger patients.
- It often starts after an acute episode of infective diarrhoea.
- The symptoms come and go over a long period, and vary from diarrhoea to constipation.
- It is associated with abdominal distension and incomplete evacuation.
- Patients often have a history of depression.

- The diagnosis is based on clinical symptoms. The majority of patients do not require investigation by colonoscopy and/or barium enemas.

Diarrhoea in HIV

Prior to HAART the causes could be split into four:
- Bacterial – *Salmonella, Shigella, Campylobacter* spp.
- Cryptosporidia and microsporidia – watery diarrhoea
- CMV colitis
- Others – IBS, *Clostridium difficile, Mycobacterium avium* complex.

However, since the introduction of HAART, both CMV and cryptosporidia/microsporidia have become uncommon. Nowadays, the side-effects of antiretroviral therapy are probably the commonest cause.

8. HYPERTENSION

Dear Colleague,
This previously healthy, 38-year-old lady felt unwell at work today with a
headache and attended my walk-in centre. I have found a blood pressure
of 230/110 mmHg and would value your opinion.

Please take a history from this patient.

Diagnoses to consider

- Secondary hypertension:
  - Endocrine hypertension:
    - primary hyperaldosteronism (Conn's syndrome)
    - Cushing's syndrome
    - phaeochromocytoma
    - acromegaly
  - Renal parenchymal or arterial disease
  - Secondary to drugs, e.g.:
    - sympathomimetics
    - combined oral contraceptive
    - NSAIDs
    - cocaine
  - Coarctation of the aorta
  - Pre-eclampsia
- Essential hypertension

Points in the history

HPC

- Features of the consequences of hypertension, e.g. heart failure, angina, stroke or TIA, renal disease (see Generic history-taking skills), headache, visual symptoms
- Features of the cause:
  - Weakness in patients with hyperaldosteronism (Conn's syndrome) to suggest hypokalaemia
  - Paroxysmal symptoms, palpitations, sweating, pallor or flushing, headache, postural hypotension, or a feeling of dread – phaeochromocytoma
  - Features to suggest acromegaly or Cushing's syndrome
  - Pulsation in the neck or throat, tired legs or intermittent claudication, angina – adult-type coarctation

- Last menstrual period
- Oedema, lethargy, haematuria, recent sore throat (streptococcal) – renal disease

PMH

- Renal infection, stones, haematuria
- Abdominal trauma – renovascular disease
- Diabetes mellitus:
  - Renal parenchymal and vascular disease
  - Secondary to Cushing's syndrome or phaeochromocytoma

Drug history

- Steroids (including inhalers, creams, lotions, drops), NSAIDs, sympathomimetics, combined contraceptive pill, appetite suppressants, carbenoxolone, monoamine oxidase inhibitors (MAOIs) (and cheese), cocaine

Social history

- Smoking – stopping smoking reduces the morbidity and mortality of hypertension to a greater extent than any antihypertensive. Malignant hypertension is more common in smokers.
- Coffee and cigarettes – together and alone, raise blood pressure.
- Alcohol – even moderate intake raises blood pressure.

Family history

- Renal disease – fibromuscular hyperplasia
- Neurofibromatosis – multiple endocrine neoplasia (type 2)

Review of systems

- Menstrual history/pregnancy

Investigations

Mandatory

- Urea and electrolytes, including bicarbonate – a metabolic alkalosis can point to potassium depletion long before the serum potassium falls from the normal range and suggests hyperaldosteronism or Cushing's syndrome

- FBC – anaemia or polycythaemia secondary to renal disease
- ESR – vasculitis or glomerulonephritis
- Glucose and lipids
- Uric acid
- Urinalysis – protein, glucose, white and red cells indicate pathology
- CXR – cardiomegaly is a sign of end-organ damage, coarctation may be revealed
- ECG – end-organ damage is revealed by LVH
- Renal ultrasound

Further investigations (in selected cases)

- Plasma renin and aldosterone
- Two 24-h urine collections and measurement of plasma catecholamines if phaeochromocytoma suspected
- Low dose dexamethasone suppression test if Cushing's syndrome suspected
- DTPA/MAG3 scan
- Nephritic screen (see p. 161)
- CT/MRI adrenals/adrenal catheter – only if supported by biochemical evidence

Management

- Admission is unnecessary unless stabilisation of blood pressure is needed acutely, e.g. malignant hypertension, with bedrest ± medication.
- Oral therapy is used unless there is encephalopathy, fitting, left ventricular failure, dissection or eclampsia.
- A sustained gradual reduction is necessary; too rapid a reduction may lead to an acute fall in cerebral perfusion pressure and thus 'watershed' strokes.
- Modifiable risk factors should be addressed before pharmacological therapy is instituted, e.g. smoking, weight, salt and alcohol intake, alongside exercise and relaxation where necessary. If these measures are successful then drugs may be avoided, although unlikely in this case.
- Attention must also be given to secondary risk factors for ischaemic heart disease, e.g. hypercholesterolaemia, diabetes mellitus (DM).
- Stop any precipitant agent.

Points of interest

- A determined search for a secondary cause must be undertaken. The prevalence of secondary hypertension depends on the diagnostic cut-off, the local referral bias and investigation routine. However, it is possible that up to 10% of unselected hypertensive patients will have Conn's syndrome.
- The treatment of Conn's syndrome depends on the aetiology: bilateral hyperplasia is best treated by medical therapy (e.g. spironolactone, amiloride); an adenoma requires surgical excision.
- The management of a phaeochromocytoma requires specialist referral. Medical therapy consists of α-blockade prior to β-blockade (unopposed β-blockade can lead to a catastrophic α-adrenergic crisis).

9. TUBERCULOSIS

A 27-year-old Asian lady is referred to the respiratory clinic by her GP. She has had a 6-week history of cough and night sweats. There is shadowing in the left upper lobe on CXR.

Please take a history from this patient.

Diagnoses to consider

- Pulmonary tuberculosis
- Lymphoma (or other malignancy)
- Sarcoidosis
- Atypical pneumonia
- Community-acquired pneumonia
- Recurrent pleural embolism (PEs)

Points in the history

HPC

- Duration of symptoms
- Is the cough productive?
- Sputum – quantity and colour
- Haemoptysis – large amount suggests TB, bronchiectasis, malignancy or aspergilloma
- Antibiotics prescribed and their effect on the symptoms
- Chest pain, often related to pleurisy
- Shortness of breath
- Weight loss
- Fevers
- Pulmonary TB – typically causes a slow onset of symptoms including productive cough, haemoptysis, weight loss and night sweats ('galloping consumption'). Consider extrapulmonary manifestations:
  - Neurological symptoms – cranial nerve palsies, meningitis, spinal cord involvement
  - Rash – e.g. lupus vulgaris, erythema nodosum
  - Adrenals – lethargy, anorexia, dizziness

- Atypical pneumonias – often associated with a dry cough:
  - *Legionella* – confusion, malaise, abdominal pain, diarrhoea and jaundice; classically caused by exposure to water coolers/air conditioning
  - *Mycoplasma* – headache, haemolytic anaemia, hepatitis and constitutional symptoms in young patients
- Sarcoidosis/lymphoma:
  - Both associated with constitutional symptoms and lymphadenopathy

PMH

- BCG vaccination or recent Mantoux/Heaf test
- Immunosuppression – HIV, immunosuppressive drugs
- Other recent infections, e.g. shingles

Drug history

- Oral contraceptive pill may be rendered ineffective as rifampicin is a powerful enzyme inducer
- Antibiotics
- Previous treatment for TB

Family history

- TB and contacts with them

Travel history

- Especially to areas of endemic TB: this includes relatives

Social history

- Occupation, crowded accommodation, contacts
- Sexual history – AIDS
- Alcohol dependency or living rough

Review of systems

Investigations

- Repeat CXR
- Sputum smear and microscopy, Gram's stain, Ziehl–Neelsen stain
- Blood cultures
- FBC, film, – haemolysis

- LFT – prior to anti-TB therapy, hepatitis (atypical infection)
- U+E – hyponatraemia (classically *Legionella*)
- Complement fixation test, rising antibody titres and urine antigen tests for atypical pneumonias
- HIV test with consent
- Mantoux test – may be negative in miliary TB and HIV
- Serum ACE
- Sputum culture for TB in Löwenstein–Jensen media – takes several weeks
- Pulmonary function tests
- Consider pleural biopsy (TB)
- CT and biopsy – lymphoma and sarcoid

Management

- Triple therapy with rifampicin, isoniazid, pyrazinamide (and ethambutol in areas where multidrug-resistant TB is common) for 2 months followed by rifampicin and isoniazid for a further 4 months.
- Side-effects:
  - Rifampicin – hepatic P450 enzyme induction; red urine, tears and sweat; diarrhoea; abnormal liver function
  - Isoniazid – peripheral neuropathy (can give concurrent pyridoxine), optic neuritis, impaired liver function and rash (erythema multiforme)
  - Pyrazinamide – arthralgia and sideroblastic anaemia; pyridoxine is often given to prevent peripheral neuropathy
  - Ethambutol – side-effects include optic neuritis and peripheral neuritis (formal colour vision testing is essential before and during treatment).
- Monitor LFTs and sputum on an outpatient basis.
- It is essential to involve the respiratory/TB nurse in the longer-term care of this patient, including contact tracing.
- TB is a notifiable disease.

Points of interest

- In much of society TB remains stigmatised and the diagnosis should be handled tactfully.
- It is essential that patients take the full antibiotic regimen as a resistant form of the disease may develop. Directly observed therapy (DOT) may be necessary.
- Regular follow-up appointments are required.

- Contacts will have to be screened.
- Rifampicin results in enzyme induction, resulting in less effective oral contraception.
- Confidentiality will need to be broken as TB is a notifiable disease.

10. LOSS OF CONSCIOUSNESS

You are referred a 28-year-old, right-handed lady by the Accident and Emergency SHO. She attended today having had an episode of loss of consciousness 2 days ago. The mother feels her daughter has not recovered completely as she is not herself. She has a headache that has been present for the last 2 weeks.

Please take a history from this patient.

Diagnoses to consider

- Seizure secondary to:
  - Mass lesion
  - Neoplasm
  - Bleed – primary or secondary to trauma
  - Infection – abscess or meningitis/encephalitis
  - Inflammation
  - Metabolic abnormality – particularly hypoglycaemia
  - Alcohol/drugs – most commonly, alcohol withdrawal
- Idiopathic/constitutional seizures
- Syncope
- Arrhythmia – SVT more likely than VT
- Vasovagal
- Left ventricular outflow obstruction – e.g. hypertrophic (obstructive) cardiomyopathy (HCM) or aortic stenosis (AS)

Points in the history

HPC

- Nature of the episode, with a witness history if necessary, to differentiate a seizure from syncope (see pp. 66,69), although the prolonged history tends against the latter.
- Define the exact duration of the illness.
- Space-occupying lesion/raised intracranial pressure – drowsiness, headache, nausea or vomiting, either preceding or proceeding from the attack.
- Localising features – motor, sensory or cerebellar symptoms. The site of origin of partial seizures may give localising value. Impairment in higher mental function or personality in frontal lobe disease.
- False localising features – diplopia from either a sixth or third cranial nerve palsy may occur.

- Infection – can result in photophobia, phonophobia or neck-stiffness.
- Hypoglycaemia – related to food.
- Trauma – can cause epilepsy in itself. Furthermore, there can be a considerable delay between the injury and presentation of a subdural haematoma.

PMH

- Intrauterine infection, birth difficulty or developmental delay
- Hypertension – malignant
- Diabetes mellitus – hypoglycaemia
- Tuberculosis, HIV – space-occupying lesion (SOL)

Drug history

- Current and past
- Steroid use (immunosuppression), diuretics – electrolyte imbalance
- Anticoagulants
- Insulin or sulphonylureas

Social history

- Alcohol use and withdrawal
- Illicit drugs
- Risk factors for HIV
- Driving
- Occupation – public-service or heavy-goods vehicle driving, operating machinery
- Exposure to flashing lights

Travel history

- Infective, e.g. histoplasmosis (USA)

Family history

- Seizures or other illness

Review of systems

Initial investigations

- ECG – evidence of structural heart disease or conduction defect
- FBC – thrombocytopenia or marker for infection
- ESR and CRP – inflammation, infection or malignancy
- U+E, LFT and bone profile – metabolic derangement
- CT with contrast or MRI brain – primary or secondary intracranial mass, intracranial haemorrhage, stroke, demyelination (only seen with MRI)
- Lumbar puncture – cerebrospinal fluid (CSF) protein, glucose, microscopy, culture, sensitivity ± electron microscopy. The presence of xanthochromia and oligoclonal bands may be important in subarachnoid haemorrhage and multiple sclerosis, respectively
- Serology for syphilis should be considered
- EEG

Further investigations

- HIV test
- *Toxoplasma* serology
- Mantoux test – can be negative in TB if patient is ill, malnourished or immunocompromised
- Cerebral lymphoma – biopsy ± CSF cytospin
- ECG, echocardiography and 24-h tape – can be helpful if diagnostic difficulty exists and a cardiac cause is suspected
- Serum ACE level if granulomatous meningitis/encephalitis is suspected
- Brain biopsy plus drainage for MC+S – may be necessary if abscess suspected

Management

- Necessarily depends on the exact nature of any disorder leading to a reduced seizure threshold.
- If any doubt exists concerning the nature of a mass lesion then tissue should be obtained for diagnosis.
- If hydrocephalus is present the pressure should be relieved.
- If an abscess is likely, treatment must be in liaison with a microbiologist and neurosurgeon. A primary focus of infection must be searched for. Drainage may be necessary if antibiotics fail.

- Bacterial and tuberculous meningitis and encephalitis need specific chemotherapy, started on the basis of clinical suspicion *immediately after* the appropriate samples for analysis have been taken.
- The diagnosis and management of idiopathic epilepsy is the realm of specialists.
- Patients with temporal lobe epilepsy should be offered surgery if two consecutive drugs fail to control seizures.
- Discuss driving restrictions.

Points of interest

- One seizure does not make one epileptic.
- Epilepsy is by definition the continuing tendency to have such seizures, even if a long interval separates such attacks.
- An EEG may support the diagnosis, but its main function is to ensure the seizures are correctly classified to enable precise treatment. The interpretation of the EEG is the domain of experts.

Driving

One should consult specific advice from *For medical practitioners at a glance guide to the current medical standards of fitness to drive*, issued by Drivers Medical Unit DVLA, Swansea: *www.dvla.gov.uk*

The following is a guide:
- After a single loss of consciousness in which investigations have **not** revealed a cause, the patient must have at least one year off driving with freedom from such attacks during this period.
- Epilepsy – once diagnosed, is defined as all events, major, minor and auras. For the purposes of the regulations, if more than one seizure occurs in a 24-hour period they are treated as a 'single event'.
- Entitlement for motor cars and motorcycles:
  - A person who has suffered an epileptic attack whilst **awake** must refrain from driving for **one** year from the date of the attack before a driving licence may be issued, or;
  - A person who has suffered an attack whilst asleep must also refrain from driving for **one** year from the attack, unless they have had an attack whilst asleep more than three years ago and have not had an awake attack since that asleep attack, and in any event, the driving of a vehicle by such a person should not be likely to cause danger to the public.
  - If the seizure is related to alcohol withdrawal the licence will be revoked or refused for a minimum of one year from the event.

- Entitlement for medium and large lorries, minibuses and buses:
  - For a licence to be issued or reissued the patient must be:
    - free of any attack for 10 years, and
    - have not required any medication to treat epilepsy, and
    - should not otherwise be a source of danger whilst driving.
- Taxi drivers:
  - Taxi drivers fall under the jurisdiction of the Public Carriage Office or the local authority and will be subject to their medical standards.

- **In all cases, it is the duty of the licence holder to notify the DVLA of the relevant details.**

11. PAIN

A 72-year-old man with known prostate cancer and bone metastases has been referred with increased pain to casualty by the Macmillan team. Co-proxamol is no longer a sufficient analgesic and the patient is now less mobile.

Please take a history from this patient.

Diagnoses to consider

- Progressive prostate cancer with:
  - Hypercalcaemia
  - Pathological fracture
  - Cord compression
  - Inability to cope at home
  - Depression

Points in the history

- First, ascertain the patient's knowledge of his condition.
- Do not assume the patient knows the diagnosis.

HPC

- Date of diagnosis, histology and PSA
- Extent of disease at diagnosis
- Treatment given and symptomatic or PSA response to treatment
- Subsequent relapses and new treatments given
- Serial PSAs over time
- Result of most recent bone scan and MRI/CT
- Pain:
  - Location – multiple sites suggests multiple metastases
  - Duration and alleviating factors (including drugs)
  - Is the pain localised or related to a fall, which would suggest a pathological fracture?
  - Previous similar symptoms related to bone metastases
- Decreased mobility:
  - Is there general weakness or weakness specifically related to the lower limbs?
  - Are there known spinal metastases?
  - Are there any sensory symptoms in the limbs, or saddle anaesthesia?
  - Presence of sphincter disturbance?

- Hypercalcaemia:
  - Increasing thirst, polyuria, nocturia
  - Confusion and fatigue
  - Constipation/abdominal pain/nausea
  - Depression

PMH

Social history

The management of this patient will rely upon a detailed social history.
- Where does he live and with whom?
- Stairs/lift, location of bedroom, toilet
- Help he gets at home (family, home help, district nurses, 'Twilight nurses', Macmillan nurses)
- Shopping, washing and cooking
- Financial support
- Is he able to leave the house and does he want to continue living there?
- Is there anything required to improve the situation at home?

Performance status is a good prognostic indicator in oncology and is commonly used.
   0 – asymptomatic
   1 – ambulatory symptoms
   2 – symptoms, but <50% of the day is spent resting
   3 – symptomatic, >50% of the day spent resting
   4 – bed-bound

Drug history

A detailed history is essential as polypharmacy is common.
- Current and previous
- Benefits vs. side-effects, e.g. constipation and confusion with opiates

Review of systems

Initial investigations

- FBC, U+E, LFT, bone profile
- Glucose
- PSA
- X-ray suspicious areas
- Bone scan

Further investigations

- If spinal cord compression is suspected, urgent imaging is required (see p. 227).

Management

Pain control

- The concept of the pain ladder is useful. One starts with simple analgesia (NSAIDs, paracetamol), moving on to compound preparations (co-dydramol), eventually moving on to opiates (e.g. morphine, diamorphine).
- Morphine should initially be given every 4 hours to titrate the dose; once a stable dose has been achieved it is switched to a 12-hour, slow-release preparation of morphine sulphate.
- Patients in pain do not become addicted; the dose may need to be increased with time due to tolerance.
- The patient should be simultaneously commenced on laxatives and antiemetics.
- Initially drowsiness is a common side-effect which subsides with time.
- Local radiotherapy is effective palliative treatment for bone metastases.
- Prostate cancer is hormone-sensitive. Gonadotrophin-releasing hormone (GnRH) analogues are effective treatment (e.g. goserelin) and have generally replaced orchidectomy. The PSA is used to measure response.
- Antiandrogens should be used for 2 weeks when starting GnRH analogues to prevent tumour flare.
- Evidence of cord compression is an emergency.

Points of interest

- Improving his quality of life is the most important issue in this patient's management.
- In PACES, discussion regarding resuscitation is usually covered in the communication skills station. However, if a good rapport has been established this discussion may be appropriate.
- PSA screening is commonly performed in the USA and is becoming more common in the UK, although its effectiveness is controversial.

12. CROHN'S DISEASE

A 45-year-old woman with known Crohn's disease has returned early to the gastroenterology clinic with increasing abdominal pain and diarrhoea.

Please take a history from this patient.

Diagnoses to consider

- Acute flare-up of Crohn's disease
- Subacute bowel obstruction due to adhesions
- Abscess or fistula
- Renal stones/appendicitis
- Colonic tumour

Points in the history

HPC

- Date of diagnosis – how and where diagnosis was made
- Investigations since – results of most recent investigations (colonoscopy, barium meal/follow-through and oesophagogastroduodenoscopy (OGD))
- Areas of GI tract affected and complications, e.g. fistulas
- Progression of disease, e.g. relapsing, remitting
- Previous flare-ups and admissions to hospital
- Previous surgery and medical treatment (e.g. steroids and aminosalicylates – rectal or oral)
- Previous response to treatment
- Abnormal urinary symptoms suggesting fistula
- LMP
- Pain:
  - Duration, location
  - Constant, intermittent or progressive
  - Alleviating factors
  - Previous similar episodes, and the cause at that time
  - Pain without diarrhoea is more suggestive of an abscess or bowel obstruction
- Diarrhoea:
  - How much diarrhoea, how often?
  - Consistency (steatorrhoea or blood)
  - Has the abdomen become larger (suggesting obstruction)?

- Is the patient able to eat and drink (if not will need admission)?
- Diarrhoea and pain is more suggestive of an acute flare-up of Crohn's disease
- Other symptoms:
  - Fevers – Crohn's disease or abscess
  - Lethargy – malabsorption or anaemia associated with chronic disease
  - Any abdominal masses – abscess or Crohn's mass
  - Non-GI manifestations:
    - eyes – conjunctivitis, anterior uveitis
    - arthropathy
    - skin lesions – erythema nodosum, pyoderma gangrenosum
    - liver disease

PMH

- Appendicitis
- Previous GI surgery unrelated to Crohn's disease

Drug history

- Steroids
- Aminosalicylates (side-effects include nausea, diarrhoea, hepatitis, pancreatitis and azoospermia)
- Azathioprine – immunosuppression, pancreatitis

Family history

- Crohn's disease

Social history

- How does the disease affect her home and occupational life?
- Family support
- Smoking – exacerbates Crohn's disease

Review of systems

Initial investigations

- FBC, U+E, LFT
- ESR, CRP (used to monitor disease activity)
- Abdominal X-ray to exclude bowel obstruction, megacolon or perforation (will also show associated calcium oxalate nephrolithiasis)

- Sigmoidoscopy and biopsy
- Stool microscopy – infection
- Pregnancy test

Further investigations

- Ultrasound scan – if there is suspicion of a collection
- Colonoscopy
- Barium studies – small bowel follow-through, enema

Management

- If a severe exacerbation (e.g. intense pain, unable to drink), the patient will need to be admitted to hospital.
- If there is evidence of bowel dilatation, liaison with the surgeons is essential.
- Treat acute pain with analgesia and hyoscine butylbromide (Buscopan).
- Chronic pain relief with opiates can be counterproductive – constipation.
- Optimise medical therapy:
  - Glucocorticosteroids (IV if severe); rectal enemas for distal disease
  - Aminosalicylates
  - Azathioprine
  - Metronidazole (useful for perianal involvement)
  - Infliximab (novel monoclonal antibody inhibiting tumour necrosis factor-α).

Points of interest

- Crohn's disease is associated with a number of extragastrointestinal manifestations:
  - Skin – erythema nodosum, pyoderma gangrenosum
  - Eyes – conjunctivitis, episcleritis, uveitis
  - Joints – asymmetrical arthropathy (ankylosing spondylitis is not related to disease activity, but is associated)
  - Liver – cholangitis, hepatitis and cirrhosis
  - Kidney – oxalate stones.
- Azathioprine and 6-mercaptopurine are not as effective in the maintenance of remission of Crohn's disease as in ulcerative colitis.
- Surgery is reserved for intestinal fistulas and obstruction that does not respond to medical therapy. Ileorectal or ileoanal anastomosis should be avoided.

13. HAEMOPTYSIS

A GP has referred a 55-year-old man who has been coughing up blood to the respiratory outpatients department.

Please take a history from this patient.

Diagnoses to consider

- Pneumonia
- Lung cancer
- Bronchiectasis
- Pulmonary emboli
- TB
- Over-anticoagulation
- Rare causes – foreign body, benign tumour, vasculitides, aspergilloma

Points in the history

HPC

- Confirm haemoptysis and not haematemesis or blood from upper respiratory tract
- Quantity of haemoptysis:
  - Moderate, i.e. a teaspoonful (5 ml) – any cause
  - Large – bronchiectasis, lung cancer, vasculitis and TB
- Duration of symptoms – if years, unlikely to be due to malignancy
- Frequency of symptoms – even a single significant episode requires investigation
- Pulmonary embolism (PE) – leg swelling, pleuritic chest pain, recent surgery/immobility/air travel, shortness of breath
- Pneumonia or TB – fevers, night sweats, sputum, contact with TB or previous chest infections
- Lung cancer – lethargy, weight loss, lymphadenopathy, bone pain and paraneoplastic symptoms
- Previous episodes of bronchiectasis or infection
- Vasculitides – fevers, joint pains, haematuria, rash

PMH

- Airways disease – longstanding shortness of breath with sputum production, associated with smoking
- Childhood respiratory infections or previous TB resulting in bronchiectasis
- Recurrent chest infections
- Thrombophilia
- Vasculitides
- Rheumatic fever – mitral stenosis

Drug history

- Anticoagulants

Family history

- First-degree relative with malignancy, especially lung cancer
- Contact with TB

Travel history

- Areas endemic with TB
- Air travel

Social history

- Occupational history (exposure to asbestos and pollution)
- A detailed social history, including family and friends, is important as the patient may become reliant on others in the future if the cause is cancer-related.
- Smoking history – calculate the number of pack-years smoked, i.e. 20 cigarettes/day for 1 year = 1 pack-year. Therefore 10/day for 20 years = 10 pack-years.

Review of systems

Initial investigations

- CXR
- FBC, ESR, CRP, U+E, LFTs, calcium
- Sputum MC+S and cytology, including acid-fast bacilli (AFB)
- Clotting, D-dimers
- Pleural fluid aspiration and biopsy (cytology, MC+S)
- Bronchoscopy and biopsy, including washings for cytology
- Urinalysis – red cell casts in vasculitides

Further investigations

- V/Q scan, and/or spiral CT scan (emboli)
- CT chest – malignancy
- High-resolution CT (fibrosis, bronchiectasis)
- Anti-GBM antibodies; ANCA
- Lung function tests
- Bone scan for staging
- PET scan (for suspected mediastinal involvement of cancer)

Management

- Depends on the underlying cause.
- Severe haemoptysis may require resuscitation.
- Although infection is the commonest cause, more sinister causes should always be considered.
- Surgery is the only treatment of any value in non-small-cell cancers, although it is suitable in only a minority of cases, due to frequent involvement of mediastinal nodes and poor lung function (requires FEV_1 of >1.5 litre for pneumonectomy).
- Chemotherapy is the treatment of choice for small-cell cancer (various regimes), but poor prognosis.
- Radiotherapy is useful for palliation of haemoptysis, bone pain from metastases and in those unfit for surgery.
- Endobronchial laser may also offer palliation.
- Early involvement of oncology multidisciplinary team (palliative care, Macmillan nursing, patient support groups).

Points of interest

- Even with an obvious mass on the CXR, one should not discuss a diagnosis of cancer without tissue histology. See communication skills (p. 273).
- While asbestos exposure predominantly causes mesothelioma, the incidence of which is increasing dramatically, there is a synergistic relationship between smoking and asbestosis and the development of bronchial carcinoma, usually adenocarcinoma.
- Asbestos-related disease may entitle patients to compensation (Industrial Injuries Act); this does not apply to pleural plaques.

Wegener's granulomatosis

- Systemic vasculitis with necrotising granulomas. Previously known as lethal midline granulomatous disease. Its prognosis has been transformed with the introduction of cyclophosphamide.
- Symptoms include nasal discharge, malaise, haemoptysis and renal failure.
- The disease is c-ANCA positive in >90% of cases and is treated with immunosuppressive therapy – IV cyclophosphamide.

Goodpasture's syndrome

- Autoimmune disease characterised by deposition of anti-GBM antibody in the alveolus and glomerulus, resulting in recurrent pulmonary haemorrhage and severe progressive glomerulonephritis.
- Diagnosis – serum anti-GBM antibodies, lung or renal biopsy.
- Treatment is with immunosuppressive therapy and plasmapheresis.
- If alveolar haemorrhage is suspected, transfer factor for carbon monoxide (T_LCO) may be increased. This can also be used to monitor the disease.

14. HIV-RELATED HEADACHE

An HIV-positive male has referred himself to casualty with a headache. His partner thinks that he has been behaving slightly bizarrely recently.

Please take a history from this patient.

Diagnoses to consider

- Cerebral toxoplasmosis
- Primary cerebral lymphoma
- HIV encephalopathy
- Progressive multifocal leucoencephalopathy (PML)
- TB meningitis
- Bacterial/cryptococcal meningitis
- Viral meningitis/encephalitis
- Intracerebral bleed
- Migraine
- Drugs

Causes are often related to the CD4 count

CD4 count (<50/mm³)	CD4 count (<200/mm³)
Primary cerebral lymphoma	Toxoplasmosis
HIV encephalopathy/PML	TB/bacterial meningitis
Cryptococcus meningitis	

Approach to the patient

- The patient should be asked if he would like his partner to be present during the consultation, as confidentiality must be maintained if requested.
- Is the patient oriented in time and space? If not, a collateral history from the partner may be necessary.
- Remember symptoms are not always related to HIV in these individuals. Common causes affecting immunocompetent patients should not be overlooked.

Points in the history

HPC

Headache:
- Sudden onset – infection, migraine or intracerebral bleed
- Progressive onset and worse in the mornings – suggests increased intracranial pressure
- HIV encephalopathy and progressive multifocal leucoencephalopathy (PML) – progressive onset associated with dementia
- Meningitis – neck stiffness, photophobia, phonophobia, fever and rash (meningococcal)
- Mass lesions (e.g. bleed, toxoplasmoma, tuberculoma, lymphoma) – focal neurology
- TB/lymphoma – constitutional symptoms (drenching night sweats, weight loss and fevers)
- Tension headache and migraine – previous similar episodes, known precipitants (e.g. cheese or red wine)

Specific points:
- Contact with cats – toxoplasmosis
- Contact with birds – *Cryptococcus* spp.
- Previous TB – respiratory symptoms, BCG and lymphadenopathy
- Feelings of déjà vu associated with herpes simplex encephalopathy – temporal lobe involvement

HIV history – (see p. 75)

PMH

- Migraine
- Sinusitis

Drug history

- Alcohol, IV drugs, cocaine and other recreational drugs

Social history

Family history

Review of systems

Investigations

- CT scan with contrast – an enhancing mass is likely to be either toxoplasmosis, lymphoma or tuberculoma (less common)
- Lumbar puncture (if CT is normal) – measure protein level, glucose, MC+S, AFBs, India ink and cytology
- FBC, U+Es, LFTs
- CD4 count and viral load
- Serum toxoplasmosis IgG titres
- CXR – TB can also cause a cerebral mass
- MRI – demonstrates all lesions of toxoplasmosis (not all are revealed by CT), and diffuse white-matter lesions of PML
- Cerebral thallium-201 scanning may be useful for distinguishing lymphoma from other causes of focal lesions, combined with polymerase chain reaction (PCR) amplification for EBV. The latter is positive in lymphoma, but negative in other causes, e.g. toxoplasmosis
- Biopsy (see below)

Management of cerebral toxoplasmosis

- HIV+ve patients with a cerebral mass are usually treated empirically for toxoplasmosis (pyrimethamine and sulfadiazine) and rescanned after a few weeks.
- If there has been no response, biopsy of the lesion may be required.
- Dexamethasone may be needed for mass effects.
- Long-term prophylaxis is required for proven cases.

Points of interest

- HIV is a retrovirus which targets T-helper (CD4) cells resulting in immunosuppression.
- AIDS is a clinical diagnosis based on the development of immunodeficiency, resulting in opportunistic disease. Not all opportunistic infections or malignancies are AIDS-defining diagnoses.

- Common diseases in HIV (normal CD4 count ~800/mm^3):

CD4 count	Disease
>200/mm^3)	Herpes simplex, herpes zoster and bacterial infections
<200/mm^3)	Non-Hodgkin's lymphoma, TB, toxoplasmosis and PCP
<50/mm^3)	CMV, MAC and primary cerebral lymphoma, progressive multifocal leucoencephalopathy

- HAART (highly active antiretroviral therapy) results in decreased viral turnover and a recovery in the CD4 count:
  - Unfortunately, the virus usually becomes resistant to the combination of drugs over time, resulting in a fall in the CD4 count and rising viral load
  - Patients who develop resistance should change their combination of HAART. Resistance testing to antiretroviral drugs can help make this decision.
- There are three main classes of drugs:
  - Nucleoside analogues, non-nucleoside analogues and protease inhibitors
  - Most patients are on triple therapy, consisting of two nucleoside analogues and either a protease inhibitor or a non-nucleoside analogue
  - Changing therapy should be performed by HIV specialists, and according to drug-resistance profiles.
- The CD4 count drops in response to increasing virus production.
- A good way of representing their interaction is using a railway train as an analogy, where the CD4 count represents the length of the track and the viral load is the speed of the train:
  - The higher the viral load, the faster the train, and therefore the quicker it comes to the end of the track
  - The lower the CD4 count, the shorter the track, and therefore the faster the train will get to the end
  - HAART initially slows down the train and often extends the length of the track.

15. ASTHMA

As the medical SHO on call, you have received this referral letter from a local GP:

Dear Colleague,
This 19-year-old lady has become increasingly breathless. She has a history of asthma and I have tried increasing the frequency of her salbutamol inhaler, but to no avail. Please see and advise.

Diagnoses to consider

Acute exacerbation of asthma due to:
- Infection
- Non-compliance with medication
- Unknown aetiology
- Exposure to allergen
- Stress
- Pneumothorax
- Pulmonary emboli
- Pneumonia

Points in the history

HPC

Prior to taking a detailed history, quickly assess for signs of life-threatening disease (inability to complete sentences, confusion, respiratory rate >25/min, hypoxia, cyanosis, hypotension and tachycardia, quiet chest).
- Questions relating to current symptoms:
  - Onset and duration of symptoms; diurnal variation
  - Consider precipitating factors – infection, contact with known allergens (e.g. cats, dust, pollen), stress, poor compliance with medication, drugs (e.g. NSAIDs)
  - Nocturnal cough
  - Discuss her normal peak expiratory flow rate (PEFR) when well, and how it has changed recently – morning dipping
  - Pneumothorax or pulmonary emboli – chest pain ± haemoptysis, recent travel
  - Atypical pneumonia – fever, cough (non-productive), confusion

- Questions related to the underlying disease:
  - When the diagnosis was made
  - Underlying stability/severity of the disease
  - Reversibility associated with therapy
  - Previous precipitating factors – stress, exercise
  - Usual treatment – home nebulisers, steroids
  - Previous exacerbations and their management
  - Previous admissions to ITU
  - Primary or secondary care of her management

PMH

- Eczema, atopy, nasal polyps
- Recent surgery

Drug history

- NSAIDs
- β-blockers
- Allergies to antibiotics
- Contraceptive pill

Travel history

- Recent air travel

Social history

- Anxiety and stress
- Smoking

Family history

- Asthma
- Clotting disorders

Review of systems

Initial investigations

- PEFR
- Pulse oximetry
- Arterial blood gases
- CXR
- FBC, U+E, CRP and ESR
- Sputum MC+S

Further investigations

- Spiral CT scan
- Lung function tests
- Serum precipitins

Management

Who to admit?

- Hypoxia, peak flow <50% of patient's normal value, tachypnoea or any signs of severe disease (see above).
- Patients with severe attacks require urgent treatment and early liaison with ITU (hypoxia <8 kPa, rising CO_2, exhaustion or hypotension).
- Patients with a history of brittle asthma should be admitted even if symptoms are mild.

Treatment of severe acute asthma

- Oxygen – high flow
- Nebulisers – β-agonists and ipratropium
- Oral steroids
- Antibiotics – if any suspicion of infection
- Hydration
- Consider oral or IV aminophylline (NB. care if on oral treatment), or IV β-agonists in unresponsive patients
- Frequent monitoring of disease activity (clinical signs, arterial gases, PEFR). Patients can deteriorate despite treatment and may require ITU admission

What if the patient is not hypoxic?

- If the initial peak flow is greater than 75% of normal, it may be possible to send these patients home with treatment modification. However, they should be observed for at least 2 hours to ensure no deterioration.
- If the initial peak flow is less than 75% of normal, doctors should err on the side of caution. Administer nebulised β-agonists and admit the patient unless there is a sustained and marked improvement in clinical condition and PEFR. If sent home, the patient should be given oral steroids and a follow-up appointment.

Points of interest

- A minority of patients have brittle asthma which can cause severe and sudden shortness of breath disease. These patients should usually be admitted to hospital.
- The management of chronic asthma should be performed in a stepwise manner (British Thoracic Society guidelines. *Thorax* 1997;52:S1–24; see: *www.brit-thoracic.org.uk*):
  - Step 1: As required, inhaled short-acting β-agonists for symptom relief
  - Step 2: Step 1 plus inhaled anti-inflammatory agents (e.g. steroids, sodium cromoglycate)
  - Step 3: Step 1 plus high-dose inhaled steroids
  - Step 4: Step 1 plus high-dose inhaled steroids, regular inhaled bronchodilators and oral theophylline
  - Step 5: Step 1 plus oral steroids.
- The efficacy of newer treatments such as leukotriene-receptor antagonists and leukotriene-synthesis inhibitors compared to established treatment requires further clinical evaluation.

16. ATRIAL FIBRILLATION

This 58-year-old gentleman was found by a surgical colleague to have an irregular pulse at a routine clinic appointment to assess his hernia. He is in otherwise good health. An ECG performed confirms atrial fibrillation. Your consultant has arranged for you to see him in his cardiology clinic today.

Please take a history from this patient.

Diagnoses to consider

Aetiology of the atrial fibrillation (AF):
- Alcohol
- Myocardial infarction
- Mitral valve disease – particularly stenosis
- Thyrotoxicosis
- Hypertension
- Pulmonary embolism
- Idiopathic – 'lone' AF
- Pneumonia
- Bronchial carcinoma

Points in the history

HPC

These relate to the aetiology:
- Chest pain, e.g. infarction, pericarditis, pulmonary embolism
- Alcohol intake
- Previous rheumatic fever
- Established ischaemic heart disease, hypertension
- Thyrotoxicosis
- Haemoptysis, weight loss – lung cancer
- Fever, cough – infection.

The arrhythmia itself:
- Palpitations, dyspnoea, dizziness, presyncope or collapses
- Likely onset of AF
- Embolic episodes, e.g. TIA, stroke, peripheral emboli.

PMH

- Bleeding diathesis
- Peptic ulcer disease
- Falls

Drug history

- Suitability for warfarin
- Other medication which might interfere with warfarin (not exhaustive), e.g. cimetidine, cholestyramine, clofibrate, amiodarone, carbamazepine, barbiturates, steroids, salicylates, azapropazone, metronidazole, antituberculous medication, erythromycin, co-trimoxazole, etc.
- Use of aspirin
- Compliance with other medications

Social history

- Alcohol intake
- Occupation and driving

Family history

Review of systems

Investigations

- ECG – diagnostic of AF, will show any associated infarction, ventricular/atrial enlargement, or the features of PE
- Echocardiography – mitral valve disease, presence of thrombus in the left atrial appendage (better seen on transoesophageal echocardiography), atrial size, wall thickness, regional hypokinesia or right ventricular strain/hypertrophy, cardiomyopathy
- CXR – cardiac size and any associated lung pathology
- FBC, ESR
- T_4, T_3 and TSH
- V/Q scan or spiral CT
- D-dimers
- LFTs including γ-GT

Management

- Oxygen
- Ensure potassium and magnesium levels are normalised
- Acutely – is the patient at high risk? (see: *www.resus.org.uk/pages/periarst.htm*)

High-risk – heart rate >150 b.p.m., ongoing chest pain or critical perfusion

- Immediate heparinisation and attempted DC cardioversion (DCC). If this fails or AF recurs, amiodarone 300 mg IV over 1 h can be given before a second attempt at DCC. A second dose of amiodarone can be give p.r.n. (as required).

Intermediate risk – heart rate 100–150 b.p.m., breathlessness

- No structural heart disease or poor perfusion:
  - If AF for >24 h is a possibility – control rate with β-blocker, verapamil, diltiazem or digoxin (do not use verapamil or diltiazem if patient is on a β-blocker). Do not attempt DCC until anticoagulated for >3 weeks
  - If AF definitely <24 h – heparinise and attempt to restore sinus rhythm (SR); use either flecainide 100–150 mg IV over 30 min, or amiodarone 300 mg over 1 h and repeated once p.r.n. Attempt DCC p.r.n.
- Structural heart disease or poor perfusion:
  - If AF >24 h a possibility – amiodarone 300 mg IV over 1 h repeated once p.r.n. Anticoagulate immediately. Do not attempt DCC until anticoagulated for >3 weeks
  - If AF definitely <24 h – heparinise and attempt DCC to restore SR. Give amiodarone 300 mg IV p.r.n. and repeat once p.r.n.

Low risk – heart rate <100 b.p.m., mild or no symptoms, good perfusion

- If AF >24 h – consider anticoagulation and DCC, if indicated, 3–4 weeks later.
- AF definitely <24 h – they can be heparinised before attempting to restore SR with amiodarone 300 mg IV over 1 h (twice p.r.n.) or flecainide 100–150 mg IV over 30 min. Attempt DCC if indicated.

Chronic management

- Avoid precipitating factors, especially alcohol, caffeine and smoking.
- AF is either paroxysmal, persistent or established. Only in the latter case is ventricular rate control with digoxin or verapamil indicated; neither drug can chemically cardiovert the AF.
- Paroxysmal AF needs cardioversion, usually by chemical means, and is most likely to succeed in recent-onset AF.
- Attempts should be made to cardiovert persistent AF. If it fails or is unsuitable, it is established AF. A dilated left atrium is a contraindication to DCC.

Points of interest

- Electrical cardioversion is chiefly useful in first attacks of AF with an identifiable cause, and in emergencies where atrial transport is vital to the maintenance of a reasonable cardiac output.
- Warfarin is superior to aspirin for thromboprophylaxis in AF (relative-risk reduction for stroke of 60–65%), and is particularly of benefit in those with hypertension (systolic >160 mmHg), poor LV function, diabetes mellitus, 75 years or over, or a previous embolus, TIA or stroke. The optimum range is an international normalised ratio (INR) of 2–3. Low-dose warfarin and aspirin is not an effective alternative; however, if warfarin is contraindicated, aspirin is beneficial.

17. WEAK LEGS

As the neurology SHO, your consultant has asked you to see the following referral:

Dear Colleague,
Thank you for seeing this 29-year-old, right-handed lady who has had weakness of her legs for the last 3 days. On examination I found the legs to be a little weak with rather brisk knee jerks.

Please take a history from this patient.

Diagnoses to consider

- Demyelination – multiple sclerosis
- Cord compression
- Hysteria/anxiety
- Myelitis
- Myopathies – associated with malignancy, thyrotoxicosis or Cushing's syndrome
- Neuropathies – e.g. Guillain–Barré, malignancy
- Intracranial mass
- Sagittal sinus thrombosis

Points in the history

HPC

- Duration of symptoms, particularly since last completely well.
- The essential diagnosis not to miss is cord compression of any description as this necessitates emergency assessment as a prelude to treatment. Pointers to this include:
  - Acute onset of weakness with sphincter disturbance and/or saddle anaesthesia
  - Known history of lymphoma, breast cancer, choriocarcinoma, primary CNS tumour or infection, e.g. TB.
- Multiple sclerosis (MS) is the most likely case in this scenario; it is characterised by lesions dissociated in space and time.
  - Previous transient diplopia, vertigo, oscillopsia or partial blindness; sexual difficulties or bladder dysfunction; prior weakness.

- Less likely diagnoses, because of the brief history and upper motor nerve signs:
  - Myopathies – symptoms of Cushing's syndrome, thyrotoxicosis or severe hypothyroidism
  - Neuropathies – diabetes mellitus, malignancy, Guillain–Barré (preceding respiratory or GI infection)
  - Myasthenia gravis – symptoms worse at end of day, ocular symptoms (NB: dyspnoea is a worrying sign in myasthenia and Guillain–Barré as it can be rapidly fatal)
  - Intracranial mass lesion – headache, loss of consciousness, focal neurology or fits
  - Myelitis – HIV, prior irradiation, vasculitis and thromboembolic tendencies (anterior spinal artery occlusion); it may occur in varicella zoster infection.

PMH

- TB
- Rheumatoid arthritis – atlantoaxial subluxation
- Operations – thymectomy
- Neck or spinal irradiation
- Diabetes mellitus
- STDs (syphilis and HIV)

Drug history

- Steroids – reactivation of TB
- Warfarin
- Diuretics – diuretic or laxative abuse may cause hypokalaemia
- Oral contraceptive pill

Sexual history

- HIV, syphilis

Social history

- Smoking and alcohol
- Occupation and nature of work, does she need to drive?
- Significant life events and temporal relationship to symptoms
- Fertility plans

Family history

Review of systems

Investigations

- Any suggestion of cord or cauda equina compression is an emergency – see spinal cord compression (p. 227).
- ESR, U+E, bone profile, LFT with γ-GT and glucose.
- TSH and T$_4$, serum vitamin B$_{12}$ level, syphilis serology, CK.
- CXR – malignancy/TB.
- MRI – the investigation of choice for MS, characteristic lesions are seen in the brain and cervical cord. Plaques of demyelination in the white matter, particularly adjacent to the lateral ventricles are readily identified. CT is less sensitive. Normal MRI (20%) does not rule out the diagnosis. Conversely, plaques may be a normal finding in some individuals.
- Evoked potentials – visual, auditory or somatosensory are sensory measures of damage in these pathways. Optic neuritis is frequently undiagnosed; a delayed visual evoked response (VER) in someone with a spastic paraparesis will provide evidence for a second lesion, favouring MS.
- Lumbar puncture – elevated CSF protein and oligoclonal IgG bands; syphilis serology is negative.

Management

- There is no curative treatment for MS.
- It is highly recommended that patients be informed of the diagnosis, when it is definite. Time must be set aside for this. In particular, open discussion, and the allaying of often misguided and ill-founded fears, is helpful.
- In those with a single lesion it is best not to discuss the possibility of MS unless specifically asked by the patient. If one must discuss the possible aetiology of an illness in front of a patient, you should avoid the term 'multiple sclerosis' until the definitive diagnosis is made; in such cases, the euphemism 'demyelinating disease' may be helpful.
- There is no method for predicting the course of the disease, but practical decisions about employment, home and future plans may need to be taken.
- Corticosteroids may accelerate recovery from acute exacerbations, but they do not protect against further relapse, nor do they affect the overall course.

- Interferon beta-1b decreases the frequency of relapses but does not prevent disability.
- About 50% of patients who have a demyelinating episode develop MS; interferon beta-1b reduces this risk by about half at 3 years.
- Muscle relaxants, e.g. baclofen, benzodiazepines or dantrolene reduce the pain and discomfort of spasticity.
- Depression is common in longstanding disease and needs aggressive treatment.
- Liaison between the GP, physiotherapist, occupational therapist and social worker is important.

Points of interest

- Cannabis is helpful for pain in some individuals; it is given sublingually in the current trials, and may soon have a licence in the UK for this indication.
- There is a striking geographical variation in the prevalence of MS:
  - It is directly proportional to the distance from the equator and is a disease of temperate climes – the prevalence in England and Wales is 60 per 100,000 and in the Shetlands, 300 per 100,000. It is a rarity at the equator. In the southern hemisphere it again becomes more common as one moves toward the South Pole.
- It is the most common neurological disorder of early adult life, but the diagnosis can be made too freely. A firm diagnosis should only be made in young adults with lesions in the central nervous system that are disseminated in space and time.
- The clinical manifestations of disease are wide as lesions can occur at any site in the CNS. There are two patterns:
  - Relapsing and remitting
  - Progressive.
- The following are common presentations:
  - Optic neuritis
  - Brainstem demyelination
  - Cervical cord demyelination.
- MS has little effect on pregnancy outcome; pregnancy has no effect on the long-term prognosis of MS.
- In this scenario, subacute combined degeneration of the cord and meningovascular syphilis are worthy of mention as causes of weak legs, not because they are likely but because they are both treatable. Motor neurone disease (see p. 232) and polymyositis (p. 355) can both present with weak legs, but are unlikely due to her age and different clinical presentation.

18. HEADACHE – 1

You are the SHO in general medicine and are referred the following patient for urgent assessment from a local GP:

Dear Doctor,
Thank you for seeing this 65-year-old lady today. She has been troubled with quite severe headaches for the past few weeks. They started rather suddenly. There is no diurnal variation. She is quite stoical and they have not responded to simple analgesia. Aside from some OA of the neck she is not normally troubled by pain. I am a little worried, as she has lost a couple of kilos in weight. I would appreciate your assistance with her further management.

Please take a history from this patient.

Diagnoses to consider

- Giant-cell arteritis
- Intracranial bleed – subarachnoid haemorrhage or subdural haematoma
- Tumours – secondary/primary, benign and malignant
- Disease of skull, sinuses and neck
- Sinusitis/mastoiditis
- Paget's disease
- Cervical osteoarthritis
- Tension headaches

Points in the history

HPC

- Exact onset and subsequent pattern of the headaches, and any associated symptoms.
- Giant-cell arteritis:
  - Short (often a few weeks) history
  - Headache may be generalised or over inflamed arteries
  - Aching, throbbing or stabbing, often worse at night
  - Jaw claudication (common), loss of taste, weakness (from internal carotid disease) can occur
  - Visual involvement, initially unilateral, is irreversible; ophthalmoplegia may occur
  - Associated malaise, fatigue, fever and depression

- Proximal muscle pain and stiffness – polymyalgia rheumatica – may improve throughout the day, such that if seen in the afternoon it may have resolved.
- Intracranial haemorrhage:
  - Subarachnoid haemorrhage (SAH) – abrupt onset, very severe, with meningism (see below)
  - Subdural haematoma – often minor trauma, if at all (none in 50%)
  - Headache is the commonest symptom; as the condition worsens, vomiting occurs
  - Fluctuating consciousness or cognition with dysphasia, weakness, incontinence, mood changes, irritability and fits may occur in chronic subdurals.
- Tumours:
  - Insidious appearance of nyctohemeral (diurnal) headache, mild initially but progressing relentlessly; the rate of progression varies with the cause and site
  - As raised pressure supervenes on stretching of intracranial contents, drowsiness, vomiting and seizures may occur
  - Consider symptoms of a primary tumour.
- Sinusitis:
  - A common complication of an upper respiratory tract infection (URTI)
  - Facial pain and tenderness, headache, nasal discharge and postnasal drip are usual.
- Mastoiditis:
  - Obvious local features
  - However, the patient may not have looked behind the ear or noticed the antecedent otitis media.
- Paget's disease:
  - Deep boring pain due to increased vascularity; or pain due to compression of nerve roots in the neck or cranial nerves.
- Cervical osteoarthritis:
  - Associated degenerative disease elsewhere; worse on movement; usually occipital pain suggesting referral from the C2 root.
- Tension headache:
  - Bilateral, 'tight band' around head with scalp tenderness, associated with stress/anxiety
  - Usually younger age group.

PMH

- Bone disease – Paget's, osteoarthritis, osteoporosis
- Malignancy
- Polycystic kidney disease (SAH)

Drug history

- Anticoagulants or antiplatelet agents
- Analgesic use
- Suitability for corticosteroids (e.g. peptic ulcer disease, DM, psychoses)

Social history

- Alcohol

Family history

Review of systems

Initial investigations

- FBC – anaemia, thrombocytosis or neutrophilia in inflammatory disease
- ESR – greatly accelerated in giant-cell arteritis (and strongly favours the diagnosis), but may be normal; more modest elevation in disseminated malignancy
- CRP – usually raised in arteritis
- U+E – disordered water balance may occur in intracranial mass lesions
- LFT and bone profile – alkaline phosphatase (ALP) raised in Paget's disease and giant-cell arteritis; coexistent bone disease is common as the population ages
- CXR – malignancy
- CT brain with contrast – if intracranial bleeding or neoplasm is suspected

Further investigations

- Temporal artery biopsy – will need to be arranged within 7 days of a suspected diagnosis of cranial arteritis, as steroid therapy will resolve the diagnostic granulomatous vasculitic changes; skip lesions may be present, thus giving a false-negative result with small biopsies.
- CK – may be helpful if there are prominent polymyalgic symptoms.
- Protein electrophoresis and urine Bence-Jones protein – essential in the differential diagnosis of an accelerated ESR.
- Blood cultures – endocarditis may mimic cranial arteritis.

Management

- Start corticosteroids immediately the diagnosis is suspected as the occurrence of visual failure may be swift. 60–100 mg prednisolone in two divided doses per day is required in patients with clear arteritic features.
- Reduce the dose on the basis of clinical course and falling or normal ESR.
- Monitor patients carefully and expect low doses (<20 mg/day) to be required for several years.
- The consequent hazards of long-term, low-dose steroids (vis-à-vis osteoporosis, insulin resistance and frank Cushing's syndrome) need attention. In particular, bone protection is usually required, e.g. bisphosphonates.

Points of interest

- Cranial arteritis and polymyalgia rheumatica are points on a spectrum of the same disease as evidenced by:
  - Similar age and sex distribution; rare before 50 years, chiefly affecting those 65–75 years of age and with a male:female ratio of 1:2
  - The myalgia and systemic features are similar
  - Similar laboratory features
  - Similar response to corticosteroids.
- Giant-cell arteritis does not reduce life expectancy.
- Corticosteroids are the only treatment; other immunosuppressive therapy has no effect.
- However, the importance of the response is perhaps overstated as many elderly patients with non-specific illness will improve on steroids.
- The initial ESR is of no use in determining disease severity, but is useful in monitoring response to therapy.
- There is no clear familial pattern to the disease, but the disease has a predilection for Caucasians, particularly Scandinavians.
- It is infrequent amongst the spouses of patients, thus arguing against an environmental cause.

19. HEADACHE – 2

You are the medical SHO on call and are referred an alert and orientated 24-year-old man who developed a severe headache today whilst in bed with his wife. He has had similar headaches from time to time over the last few years.

Please take a history from this patient.

Diagnoses to consider

- Migraine
- Subarachnoid haemorrhage
- Cluster headache/migrainous neuralgia
- Meningitis
- Coital cephalgia

Points in the history

HPC

- Headache presently?
- Exact onset of the headache and the pattern of onset:
  - Sudden or gradual?
- Any previous similar headaches?
- Subarachnoid haemorrhage:
  - Abrupt onset of devastating headache, usually occipital, which may start like a blow to the head
  - Often preceding exertion
  - Associated photo- and phonophobia with mild fever and neck stiffness because of meningeal irritation
  - Fainting and vomiting common
  - The main haemorrhage may have been heralded by warning headaches for weeks prior, as the vessel leaks.
- Migraine:
  - Paroxysmal severe, often initially unilateral headaches frequently associated with abdominal symptoms, particularly vomiting
  - Often a known precipitant
  - A prodrome may occur for several hours before the attack with fatigue, depression, elation or hunger
  - The headache builds up to its crescendo in an hour or two and usually last 12–48 hours
  - It is worsened by exertion, light and noise

- Sleep often forms an integral part of attacks – this is very uncommon in acute painful maladies
- A preceding aura defines classic migraine, which is absent in common migraine
- Visual symptoms are the most common, e.g. obscurations 'fortification spectra', frosting or scotomas, but can be sensory, motor or mood disturbance; typically last 20–40 minutes and overlap with the beginning of the headache.
- Cluster headache:
  - Very severe, daily, unilateral headaches lasting 30–120 minutes occurring in clusters lasting 4–16 weeks
  - Their severity, brevity, lack of aura or vomiting and occurrence in clusters clearly distinguish it from migraine
  - The pain is centred around one eye, which becomes red and waters profusely
  - The nose may be blocked or run
  - Restlessness betrays the frightening severity; most patients get out of bed and pace the floor
  - Alcohol and other vasodilators are common precipitants
  - Characteristically strikes at night, an hour or so after sleep, and may recur at a particular time each day, i.e. 'alarm clock headache'.
- Meningitis:
  - Fever, neck stiffness, vomiting, severe headache, rash (meningococcal) drowsiness, photo- and phonophobia may dictate consideration of this.
- Coital cephalgia:
  - May simulate subarachnoid haemorrhage
  - Occurs (more commonly in men) during or just after intercourse.

PMH

- Hypertension, diabetes mellitus, epilepsy (leaking arteriovenous malformation (AVM))

Drug history

- Analgesics taken, and benefit
- Recreational drug use
- (Combined oral contraceptive in women)

Social history

- Effect on work and home life
- Alcohol and smoking
- Stress and life events

Family history

- Migraine in 70%.
- Familial hypertension, collagen–vascular disease, thrombophilic tendency or polycystic kidney disease may all be important in SAH.

Review of systems

Investigations

- FBC – infection
- Glucose – critically ill patients with hyperglycaemia undoubtedly benefit from normalisation
- Clotting – bleeding diatheses or as a prelude to lumbar puncture
- U+E, liver and bone profile
- Blood cultures – prior to antibiotics if meningitis a possibility

Further investigations

- CT – unless the diagnosis of migraine can be made with absolute confidence it may be necessary to look for blood in the subarachnoid space. If lumbar puncture is planned it may be prudent to ensure that the intracranial pressure (ICP) is not raised.
- Low-density infarcts can occasionally be seen in severe migraine causing hemiparesis, hemianopia or aphasia, even though long-term sequelae are exceptional.
- Lumbar puncture – examine the CSF with the naked eye for blood in SAH, cloudy in meningitis, gin-clear in migraine and coital cephalgia. Xanthochromia due to altered blood pigment will be seen in SAH of 18 hours' to a few days' duration, or may point to a prior warning bleed. Perform a Gram stain urgently if meningitis suspected, together with culture/sensitivity testing (see below).
- The CSF in migraine may show a pleocytosis and raised protein level.

Management (of migraine)

- Acutely, adequate analgesia must be provided to control the pain.
- Avoidance of provoking factors – e.g. stress, alcohol, unaccustomed exercise, change in sleep pattern, bright lights, missed meals or specific foods (and menstruation and oral contraceptives) – is often neglected.

- Acute attacks of migraine:
  - Rest, dark and quiet, supplemented at the start with paracetamol or a NSAID may suffice, codeine may be required; metoclopramide may improve their efficacy by relieving gastric stasis and reducing vomiting
  - Sumatriptan can be given either orally or subcutaneously
  - Ergotamine – oral (poorly absorbed), rectal, or inhaled – effective in 50% and may be the only relief for a few patients. However, regular use can cause headaches as well as vasospasm leading to peripheral ischaemia or gangrene.
- Prophylaxis – if >2 attacks are occurring per month:
  - Propranolol and pizotifen are the commonest used; neither works for all
  - Amitriptyline, calcium-channel blockers, cyproheptadine (producing serotonin and calcium-channel blockade) and methysergide are all used – the latter only under hospital supervision for courses of 4 months (pleural, pericardial and retroperitoneal fibrosis are rare but serious side-effects resulting from prolonged use; they usually regress on withdrawal)
  - Migraine worsening before or with menstruation only occasionally responds to oestrogen implants.

Points of interest

- The availability of 24 h/day CT and local practice influences the investigation of these patients. There is a case to be made for not diagnosing migraine (nor coital cephalgia) acutely unless CT of the head and CSF examination are both normal. However, there will be times when the history is clear and one's experience allows such a diagnosis. Nevertheless, being overcautious may occasionally identify a warning bleed of an otherwise devastating SAH.
- Performing a lumbar puncture (LP) on a patient with suspected SAH or meningitis who is fully alert, has no focal signs and normal discs is probably safe and may be normal practice in some parts. Again, however, the availability of CT has led us away from performing a blind LP in most instances. Treatment for meningitis should never be delayed for an examination of the CSF.
- The earliest attack of migraine occurs before 10 years of age in one-third of patients. Over 80% have their first attack before 30 years. A diagnosis of migraine developing after 40 years must be viewed with suspicion.
- While there is a family history in two-thirds of migraineurs there is no clear Mendelian pattern of inheritance.

- The clearly neural nature of the prodrome and the lack of features attributable to vascular anatomy demonstrates that migraine is primarily of neural origin with secondary oligaemia of the microcirculation.

20. SMALL-JOINT ARTHROPATHY

As the SHO in the rheumatology clinic, you have been asked to see the following referral:

Dear Colleague,
I would be grateful if you would see this 45-year-old woman who is complaining of swelling and pain in her hand and wrists for the last 8 weeks. She had similar symptoms 6 months ago, which responded well to NSAIDs. Thanking you in anticipation.

Please take a history from this patient.

Diagnoses to consider

- Rheumatoid arthritis
- Seronegative arthritis – psoriatic (less likely in Crohn's disease, UC or Reiter's disease)
- Connective tissue diseases – SLE (less likely in polymyositis, systemic sclerosis)
- Osteoarthritis
- Septic reactive arthritis – due to *Staphylococcus* spp., *Gonococcus* spp.
- Crystal polyarthritis – gout and pseudogout

Points in the history

HPC

- Joints:
  - Site of all affected joints
  - Symmetry of involvement
  - Duration of symptoms and preceding episodes
  - Diurnal variation (morning stiffness)
  - Alleviating factors
  - Degree of functional impairment
- Systemic features:
  - Malaise
  - Weight loss
  - Rashes
  - Fever

- Specific features:
  - Rheumatoid arthritis (see also p. 371):
    - symmetrical deforming polyarthritis, classically affecting middle-aged women; consider extra-articular manifestations: eyes and mouth (dry, gritty – Sjögren's syndrome), features of neuropathy (mononeuritis multiplex, 'glove and stocking' and atlantoaxial subluxation), soft-tissue nodules, shortness of breath and chest pain (pericarditis, pleurisy, fibrosis)
  - Psoriatic:
    - characteristic rash, nail involvement and arthropathy (4 types, see p. 376)
  - SLE:
    - commonly seen in 30–40-year-old Afro-Caribbean women; non-deforming arthritis of small joints; systemic features (rashes, vasculitis, Raynaud's, renal disease, neuropsychiatric, respiratory; see p. 353)
  - Crohn's disease, UC:
    - change in bowel habit and abdominal pain
  - Reiter's disease:
    - after gastrointestinal (*Shigella*, *Salmonella*, *Yersinia* and *Campylobacter* spp.) or genitourinary infection; typically affects large joints (knees and hips), as well as conjunctivitis, urethritis, and rash (keratoderma blennorrhagica); ask specifically about previous GI or GU infections
  - Osteoarthritis:
    - commonly in hand joints or individual damaged joints in patients >60 years of age; worse in evening or with use
  - Gout:
    - typically, episodic acute pain in single joints; chronic gout occurs much later with tophi (~10–15 years later)
    - pseudogout or 'calcium pyrophosphate arthropathy' – older patients, affecting large joints, especially the knees
  - Septic reactive arthritis:
    - after systemic staphylococcal or meningococcal infection; rare

PMH

- Inflammatory bowel disease
- Autoimmune disease
- Malignancy (paraneoplastic arthropathy)
- Psoriasis
- GI infection

Drug history

- Analgesics – which ones and benefits?
- Allergies

Social history

- Occupation – cause and effects of arthritis
- Effects of arthritis on lifestyle

Family history

- Rheumatoid arthritis (10% have a family history)

Review of systems

- Reconsider the wide range of extra-articular manifestations.

Initial investigations

- X-ray affected joints – soft-tissue swelling, loss of joint space, juxta-articular osteoporosis and bone erosions
- FBC, ESR, CRP
- Rheumatoid factor, ANA, dsDNA, Scl-70
- C3 and C4 complement levels
- U+E, LFTs, bone profile
- CXR

Further investigations

- If there is any suspicion of septic or crystal arthritis, the joint must be aspirated – MC+S, crystals
- Echo, lung function tests – if systemic involvement likely
- Schirmer's test

Management (see p. 373)

Points of interest

- Reiter's syndrome is a clinical diagnosis.
- Criteria for diagnosis of rheumatoid arthritis (American Rheumatism Association (ARA)) requires four or more of:
  - Morning stiffness for >1 h – duration of >6 weeks
  - Swelling of >2 joints – duration of >6 weeks

- Swelling of wrist, metacarpophalangeal joint (MCP) or proximal interphalangeal joint (PIP) – duration of >6 weeks
- Symmetry of swollen joints – duration of >6 weeks
- Subcutaneous nodules
- Positive rheumatoid factor
- Typical radiographic features.
- Poor prognostic features:
  - Rheumatoid nodules
  - High titre of rheumatoid factor
  - Insidious onset
  - Systemic features
  - Early bone erosion
  - Persistent disease activity >12 months.

21. MALABSORPTION

A referral letter from a local GP to gastroenterology outpatients:

Dear Colleague,
Mr Parker is a 34-year-old jockey who has noticed mild weight loss and longstanding diarrhoea. His stools have been difficult to flush away and blood tests have revealed him to be folate-deficient (serum ferritin and vitamin B_{12} levels were normal). I would be grateful if you would see him and advise on his management.

Please take a history from this patient.

Diagnoses to consider

- Coeliac disease
- Crohn's disease
- Chronic pancreatitis – alcohol
- Thyrotoxicosis
- Laxative abuse
- Carcinoid syndrome
- Colonic cancer
- Whipple's disease
- Bacterial overgrowth
- Tropical sprue

Points in the history

HPC

- Amount of diarrhoea – large amounts (>300 g/24 h) suggests pathology
- Offensive and difficult to flush – small-bowel disease
- Amount of weight loss and duration
- Lethargy, associated with anaemia
- Dietary history
- Coeliac – skin lesions (dermatitis herpetiformis)
- Crohn's disease:
  - Mouth ulcers, skin lesions (erythema nodosum, pyoderma gangrenosum)
  - Abdominal pain
  - Eye involvement
  - Arthritis

- Thyrotoxicosis (see p. 405)
- Carcinoid syndrome – flushing, wheeze, abdominal pain
- Colon cancer – *per rectum* bleeding – unlikely in malabsorption (an iron deficiency would also be expected)
- Whipple's disease – arthritis, fever, neurological symptoms
- Tropical sprue – overseas travel

PMH

- Radiotherapy – radiation enteropathy
- Abdominal surgery – bacterial overgrowth
- Autoimmune disease
- Pancreatitis

Family history

- Coeliac disease (common in Ireland – HLA B8)
- Crohn's disease

Drug history

- Laxative abuse
- Thyroxine

Social history

- Alcohol history – number of units per week

Travel history

- Tropical sprue – can occur years after travel abroad (Caribbean and Asia)

Initial investigations

- FBC – anaemia, usually macrocytic
- ESR increases in Crohn's disease
- LFTs including γ-GT – low albumin level (commonly occurs in malabsorption)
- Faecal fat to confirm steatorrhoea
- Vitamin B_{12}/folate/ferritin levels (confirm deficiencies)
- T_4, T_3, TSH – thyrotoxicosis
- Antibodies to gliadin $\pm$ endomysium – coeliac disease
- Two 24-h urine 5-hydroxyindoleacetic acid (5-HIAA) levels – carcinoid tumour
- Amylase – pancreatitis
- Bone profile and vitamin D level

Further investigations

- Jejunal biopsy to confirm diagnosis of coeliac disease
- Colonoscopy/barium enema for Crohn's disease and cancer
- CT abdomen – chronic pancreatitis
- Barium studies for blind-loop syndrome

Management (coeliac disease)

- Gluten-free diet
- Dietician referral
- Patient support groups
- A repeat biopsy should be performed once the symptoms have settled

Points of interest

Coeliac disease

- The prevalence is 1/1,200 in the UK, but rises to 1/300 around Galway Bay in Ireland.
- The adverse reaction is to gliadin, a constituent of gluten which is present in wheat, barley, rye and oats.
- First-degree relatives have a 5% chance of developing the disease – HLA B8, DR3, DQW2 are implicated.
- The characteristic pathological picture is of subvillous atrophy.
- There is a small increased risk of small-bowel lymphoma and carcinoma as well as oesophageal carcinoma.
- It is associated with hyposplenism, osteomalacia and infertility.
- Dermatitis herpetiformis is a frequent skin manifestation of the disease.
- Three peaks of presentation (infancy – on introduction of gluten-containing foods; third decade – usually during pregnancy; and in the 5th decade).

Whipple's disease

- Tends to occur in men >40 years of age: the causative organism is the bacterium *Tropheryma whippelli*.
- Jejunal biopsy is required for diagnosis (stunted dilated villi with characteristic periodic acid–Schiff (PAS)-laden macrophages in the mucosa, surrounded by *T. whippelli* bacteria on electron microscopy).
- Treatment is with prolonged tetracycline or co-trimoxazole.

Small-bowel bacterial overgrowth

- The steatorrhoea is due to a failure of bile salt reabsorption, resulting in poor fat absorption.
- The terminal ileum is affected, resulting in vitamin B_{12} deficiency (serum folate is often raised).
- Fistulas, blind loops, diverticula and strictures are the most common cause, often as a result of surgery or Crohn's disease.
- Faecal fat is elevated and barium studies often reveal the nature of the pathology.
- Treatment is with low-dose, long-term antibiotics.

Vitamin deficiencies

- Folate deficiency – lack of green vegetables and diseases of the proximal ileum, e.g. coeliac disease, Whipple's disease, tropical sprue and excess alcohol intake (impaired utilisation).
- Vitamin B_{12} deficiency – lack of meat, and Crohn's disease and bacterial overgrowth.
- Iron deficiency is associated with blood loss, coeliac disease, Whipple's disease and tropical sprue.

22. NEPHROTIC SYNDROME

A patient is referred to the gastroenterology clinic from a local GP. As the SHO you are asked to see him in clinic:

Dear Doctor,
This 34-year-old man, who has been feeling non-specifically unwell has marked peripheral oedema. This has been getting progressively worse over a number of weeks. I arranged some baseline investigations which have revealed the following results: serum albumin 19 g/dl, 24-hour urine protein 4.5 g and serum creatinine 133 mmol/l (NR 60–120).

Please take a history from this patient.

Diagnoses to consider (nephrotic syndrome)

- Glomerulonephritis, especially minimal-change and membranous types:
  - Hepatitis B and C
  - Systemic vasculitides – e.g. SLE, polyarteritis nodosa (PAN)
  - HIV
  - Malaria
- Diabetes
- Allergy – bee sting
- Amyloid
- Drugs
- Malignancy

Points in the history

HPC

- Onset of the oedema
- Urinary symptoms including frequency, haematuria, pigmentation (the urine is often frothy in nephrotic syndrome)
- Constitutional symptoms (lethargy is often associated with renal failure)
- Questions relating to the cause:
  - Glomerulonephritis:
    - autoimmune disease – joint pain, rash, eye symptoms
    - recent bacterial infection – streptococcal
    - risk factors for hepatitis B and C or episodes of jaundice
    - recent travel and fevers – malaria

- Malignancy (particularly myeloma) – weight loss, lymphadenopathy
- Diabetes – longstanding or new onset (thirst, polyuria, nocturia and weight loss)
- Amyloid – waxy skin, altered bowel habit
- Questions relating to complications of the disease:
  - Venous thrombosis – occlusion of leg, neck and hepatic veins
  - Pneumococcal sepsis due to loss of immunoglobulins
  - Symptoms of renal failure – lethargy, urinary symptoms

PMH

- Diabetes
- Malignancy
- Autoimmune disease

Drug history

- Penicillamine
- Gold
- Allergies – nuts and bee stings

Social history

- Alcohol

Travel history

- Areas of endemic malaria

Initial investigations

- 24-hour protein level
- EDTA (ethylenediaminetetraacetic acid) scan for GFR
- FBC, ESR – myeloma and glomerulonephritides
- CRP – not raised in myeloma
- U+E, calcium, LFTs
- Glucose and HBAic
- Hepatitis B + C serology; HIV test
- ASO titre and throat swab
- Urine microscopy for red-cell casts – glomerulonephritis
- Serum electrophoresis and immunoglobulins; spot urine for Bence-Jones protein – myeloma
- Rectal biopsy – amyloid
- CXR

- Cholesterol – increased LDL, normal HDL in nephrotic syndrome
- ANA, dsDNA, C3, C4

Further investigations

- Renal biopsy
- Arteriography – PAN

Management

- Treat the underlying cause
- Dietary sodium restriction
- Diuretics
- Prophylactic antibiotics against streptococcal infections
- Anticoagulation, if patient is immobile
- High protein diet ± intravenous immunoglobulins

Points of interest

Amyloid

- Heterogeneous collection of disorders characterised by protein deposition in pleated sheets:
  - AA – associated with chronic inflammatory disease. 95% of patients present with proteinuria. The median survival is 5 years
  - AL – usually associated with myeloma. It tends to affect other organs as well as the kidneys. The median survival is 10 months.
- Other features of amyloid include waxy skin, hepatosplenomegaly, restrictive cardiomyopathy and altered bowel habit.
- Diagnosis is by rectal biopsy – characteristic birefringence on microscopy of biopsy.

Minimal-change glomerulonephritis

- Unknown aetiology, occurs in the young and does not usually lead to renal failure.

Membranous glomerulonephritis

- Associated with SLE, malignancy, malaria and penicillamine.
- Commonly causes endstage renal failure. Usually occurs in adults.

STATION 3

The Cardiovascular
and Neurological
Examinations

The Cardiovascular Examination

Contrary to the belief of most candidates, the examination of the cardio-vascular system does not end with auscultation of the precordium or the lung bases, but must include, if appropriate, relevant examination of the abdomen, lower limbs, urine and other areas. In PACES there is plenty of time to complete the examination; even though in the arena of the examination the majority of cases will focus on valvular pathology, one must also look broadly at the patient.

APPROACH TO THE PATIENT

- Introduce yourself.
- Position the patient correctly.
- Expose the patient from the waist up; a sheet can cover the chest initially if appropriate, but will have to be completely removed for a general inspection.
- Position the patient at 45°, with the head resting on enough pillows to relax the sternomastoids.
- Ask if they are at all in pain and ensure they are comfortable.
- Explain what you want to do briefly: 'I am just going to feel your pulse and listen to your heart; is that alright?' may suffice.

GENERAL APPEARANCE

- Mitral facies – pulmonary hypertension, classically mitral stenosis (MS)
- Central cyanosis
- Differential cyanosis – patent ductus arteriosus and pulmonary hypertension
- Pallor
- Dyspnoea
- Accessory muscles of respiration
- Down's syndrome – ventricular septal defect (VSD)
- Turner's syndrome – coarctation, bicuspid aortic valve (AV), aortic stenosis (AS)
- Noonan's syndrome – pulmonary stenosis (PS)
- Teeth must be examined in all cases – infective endocarditis

Hands

Check the following:
- Dilated veins and palmar erythema in CO_2 retention
- Temperature – cool peripheries associated with poor flow; hyperdynamic circulation
- Peripheral cyanosis
- Clubbing – cyanotic congenital heart disease; infective endocarditis; atrial myxoma (very rare)
- Capillary pulsation – aortic regurgitation (AR), patent ductus arteriosus (PDA)
- Osler's nodes, Janeway lesions, splinter haemorrhages – infective endocarditis
- Nail-fold telangiectases – collagen vascular disease
- Arachnodactyly – Marfan's syndrome
- Xanthomas – hyperlipidaemia.

Radial and brachial pulses

- Check the rate, rhythm and synchronicity.
- Look for radiofemoral delay.
- If the pulse is chaotic, it is usually AF.
- Character – the only aspect of character that can be reliably assessed at these pulses is a collapsing or 'waterhammer' pulse.
- Look over the brachial artery for scars from previous angiography.
- Ask to measure the blood pressure.

Jugular venous pulse

- It has three waves ('a', 'c' and 'v'), and two descents ('x' and 'y').
- By convention, it is measured with the patient lying at 45° when it is often visible just above the clavicle.
- The neck must be fully supported by pillows so the sternomastoid muscles are fully relaxed.
- The head should be turned slightly to the side and a light shone obliquely across the neck to maximise the shadows of venous pulsations.
- It is measured in vertical height from the angle of Louis (sternal angle), and is normally 3–5 cm (of water/blood).
- Alteration of the patient's position does not affect the *height* of the JVP, but will alter its *position*.

- This helps to differentiate it from the carotid pulse, along with its:
  - Site
  - Double waveform
  - Ability to be compressed and obliterated
  - Presence of the hepatojugular reflux.
- If one cannot see the waveform, the vessel may be kinked and thus one cannot reliably use the JVP as a right atrium manometer.

Abnormal JVP

- Raised in fluid overload – commonly heart failure, but also in pregnancy and overenthusiastic intravenous fluid administration
- Giant 'v' waves – tricuspid regurgitation (TR)
- No 'a' waves – AF
- Inspiratory filling (Kussmaul's sign) – pericardial constriction (e.g. tuberculous pericarditis), tamponade (e.g. renal failure, post-MI, viral pericarditis, malignancy) and severe asthma
- Cannon waves – atrio-ventricular dissociation, commonly complete heart block and also ventricular tachycardia (VT)

Carotid pulse

Three components:
- Percussion wave – the shock wave transmitted up the elastic wall of the artery
- Tidal wave – the forward-moving column of blood follows the percussion wave and is normally palpable separately
- Dicrotic notch – occurs with aortic valve closure

Abnormal carotid pulse

- Large volume collapsing – very brisk upstroke then rapid diastolic run-off from the aorta – AR, PDA, thyrotoxicosis, pregnancy and sepsis/fever
- Anacrotic – slow-rising with delayed percussion wave and sometimes a palpable judder (the anacrotic notch) on the upstroke, in AS
- Bisferiens – mixed aortic valve disease with significant regurgitation
- Judder on the upstroke – the percussion wave is followed by a pronounced tidal wave, thus a jerky pulse, in hypertrophic cardiomyopathy (HCM)
- Alternans – alternating large and small beats in very poor LV function, e.g. failure, AS, dilated cardiomyopathy

PALPATION

Apex beat and cardiac pulsations

- Displaced but not enlarged in pectus excavatum or scoliosis.
- Normally located at the fifth intercostal space in the mid-clavicular line; measure it from the angle of Louis; palpable but does not lift the finger off the chest.
- If abnormal decide whether it is:
  - Volume-loaded – mitral regurgitation (MR), aortic regurgitation (AR) or atrial septal defect (ASD)
  - Hyperdynamic, laterally displaced – 'thrusting'
  - Pressure-loaded – AS, hypertension (HT) or HCM as long as the LV function is good
  - Forceful, minimally displaced – 'heaving'
  - Lateral and diffuse – left ventricular failure (LVF), dilated cardiomyopathy (DCM)
  - Double-impulse (palpable atrial systole) – HCM.
- Lay the flat of the hand along the left sternal edge to feel for the sustained pressure of a left parasternal heave – RV hypertrophy of any cause, e.g. pulmonary stenosis (PS), cor pulmonale, ASD.
- Palpate each valve area in turn with the flat of the fingers, for palpable heart sounds and thrills:
  - Palpable in forceful closure
  - S_1 – MS
  - P_2 – pulmonary HT
  - S_1 and S_2 – thin patients with tachycardia.

Thrills

- Aortic area – AS
- Left sternal edge – VSD or HCM
- Apex – MR (often due to ruptured chords)
- Pulmonary area – PS
- Subclavicular area – subclavian artery stenosis
- Occasionally a diastolic thrill:
  - At the apex in MS
  - Left sternal edge in AR

AUSCULTATION

Listen to each valve area in turn and then the carotids.[1]

Heart sounds

- The valve sounds are all low frequency in health, best heard with the bell of the stethoscope.
- Any added sounds – murmurs, snaps, clicks or rubs.
- Radiation from the valve areas.
- M_1 and A_2 are louder than and precede T_1 and P_2; the split is wider in inspiration.
- The split is reversed in AS, left bundle-branch block (LBBB) (e.g. IHD), RV pacing.
- S_2 is single in a large VSD; fixed and wide in an ASD.
- S_3 – pathological over 30 years of age, when due to rapid filling, e.g. MR or VSD, or a dilated LV with a high LV end-diastolic pressure (LVEDP), e.g. post-MI (associated with a poor prognosis) or DCM.
- S_4 – occurring at the end of diastole in HT, AS, PS, HCM or after an MI; it disappears in AF.

Murmurs

- Innocent – ejection systolic, between LSE and PV, occasionally apical; no thrill, added sounds, or cardiomegaly; normal ECG, CXR and echo.
- Pathological:
  - Organic – valvular, subvalvular
  - Functional – dilated valve ring or increased flow.
- Individual murmurs are discussed in their relevant sections.
- Loudness can be graded as 1–4 for diastolic murmurs and 1–6 for systolic or, more helpfully, 'just audible', 'soft', 'moderate' and 'loud'.
- Classify as to:
  - Site,
  - Radiation,
  - Timing, and
  - Behaviour with respect to respiration and movement and effort if necessary.

---

1 Candidates should understand there are a number of acceptable routines in auscultation of the heart. Examiners will often have their own preference and may ask you to explain your method. However, as long as you are clear as to why you are following your particular routine, you are unlikely to be penalised.

Lung bases

- Need to be examined for oedema.

ABDOMEN

An examination of the cardiovascular system in PACES may well stop at the lung bases. However, it may be necessary to examine for:
- Hepatomegaly – if TR is suspected
- Splenomegaly – if infective endocarditis is a possibility
- Abdominal aortic aneurysm – elderly patient, but unlikely to be the focus of the case
- Renal bruits – if macrovascular disease suspected.

PERIPHERY

- Palpate the peripheral pulses.
- Examine for peripheral oedema (firm pressure for up to 30 seconds against the tibia 6 cm above the medial malleolus).

DIP THE URINE

STATION

Cardiovascular Scenarios

1. MITRAL STENOSIS

Points in the examination

- Left thoracotomy scar
- Malar flush (mitral facies)
- Chaotic ('completely irregular' or 'irregularly irregular' are alternative terms) low-volume pulse
- JVP normal height, prominent 'v' wave (if tricuspid regurgitation secondary to right ventricular hypertrophy (RVH))
- Undisplaced tapping apex; left parasternal heave (if RVH)
- Loud S_1, opening snap, mid- to late-diastolic, rumbling, low-frequency murmur, at the apex, best heard in the left lateral position, radiating to the axilla; accentuated by exertion

Severe disease

- Short duration between S_1 and opening snap
- Longer duration of diastolic murmur
- Severity of dyspnoea

Aetiology

- Rheumatic valvular disease is by far the commonest cause – Lancefield Group-A streptococci cell wall antigens crossreact with the heart valve structural glycoproteins causing inflammation and then commissural fusion
- Non-rheumatic disease – very rare, e.g.:
  - Congenital – mucopolysaccharidoses
  - Endomyocardial fibroelastosis
  - Malignant carcinoid

Differential diagnosis

- Inflow obstruction:
  - Left atrial (LA) myxoma
  - Ball-valve thrombus
- Austin Flint murmur – associated with aortic regurgitation (AR), collapsing pulse, volume-loaded ventricle, and early diastolic murmur (EDM) at the left sternal edge (LSE)

Symptoms

- Dyspnoea on exertion, orthopnoea and PND as secondary pulmonary hypertension develops; pulmonary oedema may be precipitated by AF, pregnancy, exercise, a chest infection or anaesthesia
- Fatigue – because of the low cardiac output in moderate to severe stenosis
- Haemoptysis:
  - Alveolar haemorrhage
  - Bronchial vein rupture
  - Pulmonary infarction because of the low cardiac output and immobility
  - Bloody sputum, with chronic bronchitis due to bronchial oedema
- Systemic emboli occur in 20–30% of cases, e.g. cerebral, mesenteric, saddle or iliofemoral
- Chest pain – RVH with normal coronaries
- Palpitations and paroxysmal AF
- Right heart failure with TR and hepatic angina, ascites and oedema
- Dysphagia – from left atrial enlargement
- Infective endocarditis is unusual

Investigations

- ECG – AF, or if in sinus rhythm P mitrale; RVH; low voltage in V1; progressive right ventricular hypertrophy (RAD)
- CXR – splaying of the carina; double right heart border (enlarged left atrium); convex left heart border
- Echocardiography – necessary for differential diagnosis and to calculate the valve area
- Catheter – not initially, unless previous valvotomy, other valve disease, prior to surgery, angina or valve calcification on the CXR

Management

- Medications
- Digoxin ± verapamil or β-blocker – if AF
- Diuretics
- Warfarin if previous emboli; prosthetic mitral valve; low output with right heart failure; AF; moderate MS and no appendectomy
- The decision to intervene is based upon symptoms (NYHA grades 3–4) or a valve area of <1 cm^2; options are valvuloplasty or surgery (closed or open commissurotomy or MV replacement)

2. MITRAL REGURGITATION

Points in the examination

- Chaotic, small-volume pulse present.
- Apex is laterally displaced and hyperdynamic.
- Left parasternal heave is present– if RVH.
- S_1 is soft; A_2–P_2 may be wide; P_2 is loud if there is pulmonary hypertension, S_3 (this indicates rapid ventricular filling and thus negates any significant mitral stenosis).
- Apical blowing pansystolic murmur, going through S_2, and radiating to the axilla.
- If there is coexistent mitral stenosis then the balance of the two lesions dictates the signs.
- The loudness of the murmur is of no significance.
- Murmurs at the LSE may be MR.
- The murmur may be a pansystolic murmur (PSM), late systolic or ejection systolic ESM.

Severe disease

- A soft S_1 and an S_3
- Degree of displacement of apex
- Dyspnoea

Symptoms

- The above examination describes chronic MR (which is the most likely exam case) – the left atrium is large and compliant and thus the lesion can be well tolerated.
- Symptoms are similar to MS with chronic dyspnoea and fatigue, but haemoptysis and emboli are less common. However, infective endocarditis is more common.
- In acute MR the LA is small, and the pulmonary venous pressure rises rapidly resulting in gross pulmonary oedema. It is very poorly tolerated and may need valve replacement as an emergency. It will obviously not be seen in the examination:
  - The patient is often in SR, with an apical thrill because of chordal rupture; the murmur is often ejection systolic
  - Causes are posterior papillary muscle dysfunction in an inferior MI, or infective endocarditis.

Differential diagnosis

- AS – regular, slow-rising pulse, pressure-loaded apex and ESM in the aortic area
- Mitral valve prolapse (MVP) – mid-systolic click; may have a late systolic murmur
- HCM – jerky pulse; double, forceful pressure-loaded apex and ESM at the LSE
- VSD – often a thrill and a PSM, but both maximal at the LSE
- TR – RV heave, murmur loudest at the LSE in inspiration and giant 'cv' waves in the JVP
- ASD – right heart signs predominate, pulmonary ESM, but P_2 does not move on inspiration (fixed splitting)

Aetiology

Varied, and includes all structures involved in valvular function:
- Functional:
  - Commonly secondary to dilatation of the mitral valve annulus, either an ischaemic left ventricle or a dilated cardiomyopathy
  - In elderly females > males, calcification of the annulus (lateral CXR) is seen; this can extend to involve the cusps, causing MR or it may be benign. It is associated with diabetes mellitus and Paget's disease, and doubles the relative risk of embolic stroke.
- Structural:
  - Valvular regurgitation is caused by rheumatic fever or infective endocarditis.
- MV prolapse:
  - Mitral valve prolapse forms a whole spectrum of disease, from an asymptomatic patient with a mid-systolic click to one with severe MR with chordal rupture. If there is a murmur then infective endocarditis prophylaxis is necessary
  - Chordal rupture may be idiopathic or associated with the floppy valve because of myxomatous degeneration, or may be secondary to ischaemia
  - Posterior papillary muscle dysfunction commonly occurs in an inferior MI, whereas anterior papillary muscle dysfunction, occurring in large anterior MIs with right coronary artery (RCA) involvement, is much rarer.

Investigations

- ECG – AF; SR with P mitrale; LVH ± RVH
- Echo – will show LA size and rapid filling; Doppler will show the size and site of the MR jet
- CXR – enlarged LV; enlarged LA if chronic; MV calcification; Kerley B lines and pulmonary venous congestion
- Catheter – this is necessary to confirm the diagnosis and assess the other valves, the LV and coronaries. The LA/pulmonary wedge v wave gives a measure of severity

Management

- AF is treated with digoxin (see p. 137).
- Warfarin is withheld unless there is a history of emboli, prosthetic MVR, or coexistent MS with a low cardiac output.
- Diuretics and nitrates decrease pulmonary venous congestion and LV preload.
- Afterload reduction can abolish MR, e.g. ACE inhibitors, angiotensin-II blockers.
- Acute MR is managed as cardiogenic shock – sodium nitroprusside reduces afterload.
- Consider infective endocarditis as a consequence or a cause.
- Surgery for MVR is less successful than for MS.
- Necessary in acute MR with chordal rupture or postinfarct MR – as an emergency.
- Consider surgery for chronic MR before the LV function declines irreversibly – NYHA 3 or 4, or NYHA 2 and LV enlargement on CXR, or increasing dyspnoea.

Prognosis

- If the LV is preserved, it is well tolerated. 60% of patients with chronic MR are alive at 10 years. Prognosis depends on the LV function.
  - Poor prognostic features:
    - symptomatic history of <1 year
    - AF
    - >60 years of age
    - LVEF <50%, dilated LV
    - Echo LV size at end-systole >5 cm, end-diastole >7 cm.

3. AORTIC STENOSIS

Points in the examination

- Regular anacrotic (slow-rising with a judder) pulse.
- The carotids may be difficult to palpate in severe disease.
- Narrow pulse pressure.
- JVP normal.
- Minimally displaced pressure-loaded apex.
- Harsh crescendo–decrescendo murmur in the aortic area, radiating to carotids.
- If the valve is bicuspid and mobile, S_1 is soft, followed by an ejection click before the murmur.
- If the valve is rheumatic and calcified, or the patient is old with a calcified valve, there is no ejection click, the murmur is harsh, but S_2 is quiet, and there may follow an early diastolic murmur of aortic regurgitation.

Severe disease

- S_4 may be present in a young patient
- Reversed S_2
- Pulsus alternans
- Aortic thrill
- Displaced apex (associated cardiac failure)

Aetiology

- Either valvar, subvalvar or supravalvar
- Valvar stenosis – commonest:
  - Congenital in 7%, M:F 4:1; bicuspid aortic valves are present in 1% of the population (one-third AS, one-third mixed AV disease and one-third normal); it is the commonest cause of AS in the 40–60-year age group
  - Inflammatory – rheumatic fever causing AS and AR
  - Arteriosclerosis in type IIa hypercholesterolaemia; gross atheroma can involve the aortic wall, the major arteries, coronary arteries and aortic valve
- Subvalvar – discrete fibromuscular ring, HCM

- Supravalvar – a constricting ring of fibrous tissue at the upper margin of the sinus of Valsalva – associated with Williams' syndrome (hypercalcaemia, giant 'a' wave in JVP, PA stenosis – RVH, PA thrill, elfin facies)

Symptoms

Left ventricular hypertrophy occurs with a compensatory enlargement of the coronary circulation. There is a relatively fixed cardiac output, and thus the heart is at its maximum output at rest.

- Angina – the increased muscle mass and increased pressure in the heart muscle, in both systole and diastole, increase oxygen demand while decreasing supply. Valvar calcification can extend to the coronary ostia.
- Dyspnoea – the increased pressure within the LV increases further with exercise.
- Paroxysmal nocturnal dyspnoea and orthopnoea supervene as the LV function deteriorates.
- Giddiness and syncope – on exertion, the relatively fixed cardiac output cannot increase further.
- Sudden death can occur.
- Emboli – can arise from calcified valve.
- Symptoms of infective endocarditis can be seen.

Differential diagnosis

- Mitral valve prolapse (see p. 177)
- VSD (very small) – thrill and pansystolic murmur at left sternal edge
- HCM (see p. 196)

Investigations

- ECG:
    - SR, if in AF suspect MV disease or previous MI
    - P mitrale with a negative P wave in V1 because of the high LVEDP
    - LVH ± strain
    - Left axis deviation (LAD), left anterior hemiblock (LAHB)
    - LBBB or CHB (with calcification of the valve ring in 5%)
- CXR:
    - LVH
    - Calcification of the valve if patient >40 years of age; on lateral views the calcification is above and lateral to the oblique fissure
    - Poststenotic dilatation of the aorta
    - Pulmonary oedema and LVF

- Echo:
  - Bicuspid valve
  - Calcification
  - LVH and function
  - AR
  - Gradient assessment
- Catheter:
  - Gradient
  - LV function
  - Coronary circulation
  - Aortic root size

Management

Medical

- Nitrates and ACE inhibitors should be avoided as they increase the gradient across the valve (reduce afterload).

Surgery

- In adults, valve replacement is required once they become symptomatic. Valvuloplasty offers limited benefit in adults.
- The average survival (without surgery) once symptoms of angina/syncope occur is 2–3 years in patients with angina/syncope, and 1–2 years in heart failure without surgery.
- Surgery is often recommended if the gradient is severe (e.g. 50–70 mmHg), but is not an absolute indication.
- The mortality of AV surgery is <5%. If coronary disease or LVF is present it rises to 10–20%.

Points of interest

- Whether aortic sclerosis is a separate pathological entity from aortic stenosis remains controversial.
- In >60-year-olds, senile calcification of a tricuspid AV often occurs, but does not result in left ventricular outflow obstruction.
- The character of the pulse remains normal, with no ejection click; S_2 is normal and the murmur is localised.

4. AORTIC REGURGITATION

Points in the examination

A wealth of eponyms are associated with aortic regurgitation, mostly from the days of quaternary syphilitic aortic dilatation.
- Visible nail-bed capillary pulsations (Quincke's sign).
- Regular tachycardia (the regurgitant jet is reduced by shortening diastole).
- Full-volume collapsing ('waterhammer') pulse (unless the LV is failing).
- Wide pulse pressure.
- Bobbing head (De Musset's sign).
- Visible carotid pulsations (Corrigan's sign).
- Carotid pulse has a rapid upstroke with no dicrotic notch; if the stroke volume is large there may be a judder.
- Apex displaced inferolaterally and is hyperdynamic.
- Heart sounds are normal.
- Short, early, blowing (decrescendo), diastolic murmur at the left sternal edge with the patient sitting forward and breath held in expiration, listening with the diaphragm; there is often a shorter systolic flow murmur across the aortic valve.

Severe disease

- As the regurgitation becomes more severe, the length of the murmur increases. Listening with the bell at the apex with the patient in the left lateral position reveals a rumbling, low-pitched, mid-diastolic murmur, as the regurgitant jet causes fluttering of the anterior mitral valve leaflet (Austin Flint murmur).
- As the regurgitation becomes still more severe and the left ventricular diastolic pressure increases, the mitral valve closes prematurely (preventing forward flow) and thus S_1 is soft, and the Austin Flint murmur is abolished. The diastolic murmur becomes full length, A_2 is inaudible and P_2 is obscured.
- Duroziez's sign – this is an audible 'to and fro' murmur at the femoral artery.
- Traube's sign – gives 'pistol shot' femorals.

Aetiology

- Primary disease of the valve:
  - Congenital valve lesions
  - Connective tissue laxity:
    - Marfan's or Hurler's syndrome
- Aortic root disease with dilatation and stretching of the valve ring:
  - Hypertensive root dilatation
  - Dissection
- Secondary valve disease:
  - Rheumatic fever
  - Infective endocarditis
  - Both seropositive (rheumatoid arthritis) and seronegative arthritides (ankylosing spondylitis, Reiter's disease)
  - SLE
  - Syphilis – quaternary

Differential diagnosis

- Pulmonary regurgitation – correction of Fallot's tetralogy or a postpulmonary valvotomy; Graham Steell murmur secondary to pulmonary hypertension in mitral valve disease
- PDA – continuous machinery murmur usually loudest in 2nd left intercostal space

Symptoms

- Dyspnoea is the main symptom.
- Angina and syncope are much less common than in AS.
- It can be well tolerated if gradual compensation occurs.
- Conversely, if the onset is rapid (e.g. dissection or infective endocarditis), then LVF or CCF can rapidly supervene.

Investigations

- ECG:
  - LVH
  - ST depression and T-wave inversion occur as the condition deteriorates

- CXR:
  - Aortic valve calcification is rare in pure AR
  - LVH
  - The aortic arch may be prominent in hypertension or dissection, or aneurysmal in Marfan's or syphilis (Jaccoud's sign where the aorta is seen in the suprasternal notch); pulmonary venous congestion or oedema – severe disease
- Echo:
  - LV function and dimensions
  - Aortic valve thickening or vegetations
  - Fluttering of the anterior mitral valve leaflet with prominent mitral valve closure
  - Rarely, one may see a dilated aortic root with a double wall in dissection, or a flail aortic leaflet prolapsing into the LV outflow tract
- Catheter – to document:
  - Severity of the regurgitation
  - Anatomy of the aortic root
  - LV function
  - Coronary artery and ostial anatomy
  - Other valve disease
- Syphilis serology
- ANA/Rheumatoid factor
- Sacroiliac XR, HLA B27 haplotype

Management

- Surgery should be performed before heart failure develops.
- Consider if:
  - Enlarging heart on CXR
  - Pulse pressure >100 mmHg
  - ECG deteriorating with lateral T-wave inversion
  - 65% of patients with all three of the above will develop CCF or die within 3 years
  - Postinfective endocarditis not responding to medical management.
- Medical management is the treatment of heart failure and endocarditis prophylaxis.

5. IRREGULAR PULSE/ATRIAL FIBRILLATION

Points in the examination

- Pulse is chaotic both in rhythm and volume ('irregularly irregular').
- Radial rate less than apical, 'pulse deficit'.
- JVP – No 'a' wave.
- Apex – normal unless other disease, e.g. mitral stenosis.
- Auscultation – S_1 varies in intensity and S_2 is normal.
- Consider the aetiology – e.g. features of mitral valve disease or thyrotoxicosis.

Aetiology

- Ischaemic heart disease
- Mitral valve disease (especially stenosis)
- Hyperthyroidism
- Hypertension
- Pulmonary embolism
- Cardiomyopathies
- Alcohol
- Constrictive pericarditis
- Sick-sinus syndrome
- Lung pathology, e.g. carcinoma, pneumonia

Symptoms

- Usually none
- Palpitations – especially if paroxysmal
- Fatigue and dyspnoea
- Presyncope, dizziness
- Embolic symptoms – cf. mitral stenosis
- Of underlying cause

Differential diagnosis

- Ectopic beats – atrial or ventricular. Unifocal ectopics have a constant compensatory pause after the beat. Dropped beats are followed by a normal RR interval. Multifocal ectopics can result in a truly chaotic pulse.
- Wenkenbach AV block has a progressively lengthening RR interval, followed by a dropped beat; it is not chaotic.
- Sinus arrhythmia.

Investigations

- ECG – chaotic baseline and absence of P waves
- CXR – cardiac size and lung disease
- Electrolytes – particularly K^+ and Ca^{2+} (high or low), hypomagnesaemia, acidosis (metabolic or respiratory).
- Arterial blood gases (ABGs) – hypoxia and acidosis
- Free T_4/T_3 and TSH
- Echo – valve disease, cardiomyopathy, hypertrophy; indication for anticoagulation – chamber size or thrombus
- 24-h tape – may be necessary if paroxysmal
- An exercise tolerance test (ETT) may be necessary rarely in the young patient with exercise-induced AF

Management (see p. 137)

- Treat the underlying cause.
- Is this paroxysmal, persistent or established AF?
- Does the patient warrant anticoagulation?
- In paroxysmal or persistent AF the aim is cardioversion to, and then maintenance of, sinus rhythm; if this is unattainable, aim to minimise the duration and frequency of AF.
- Atrial systole may contribute up to 25% of cardiac output by increasing the LVEDV, and may be symptomatically critical in patients with a poor LV.
- Cardioversion is either chemical or electrical.
- In established AF the aim is rate control – digoxin ± verapamil
- Warfarin is the anticoagulant of choice, to give an INR between 2.0 and 3.0.

6. VENTRICULOSEPTAL DEFECT

Points in the examination

If very small

- Pulse – normal rate, rhythm and character
- Apex – normal and no thrills
- Heart sounds – normal
- Loud, early ejection systolic murmur (maladie de Roger) at LSE
- The differential diagnosis includes mild AS or PS

If small

- Apex – may be normal or reflect slight LV hypertrophy
- Thrill – at the LSE
- S_2 splits on inspiration but A_2 is obscured by the murmur, which is a loud pansystolic murmur at the LSE radiating to the apex and the pulmonary artery
- The differential diagnosis includes MR, TR, HCM and pulmonary stenosis

As the VSD becomes larger

- Both left and right ventricular hypertrophy occur and the pulmonary arteries may become palpable.
- Thrill – remains, but this and the murmur become softer. The jet velocity of the VSD and the pressure gradient between the ventricles is smaller, the larger the defect.
- As pulmonary hypertension becomes prominent the murmur may disappear as the ventricular pressures equalise.
- Eventually Eisenmenger's complex (a right-to-left shunt) may develop (see Eisenmenger's syndrome, p. 190).

Aetiology

Congenital

VSD as integral part of syndrome
Fallot's tetralogy
Double-outlet right ventricle
Truncus arteriosus

VSD associated with syndrome
Tricuspid atresia
Pulmonary atresia
Transposition of the great arteries
Coarctation

Acquired

Post-myocardial infarction

Differential diagnosis

- Mitral valve regurgitation
- AS
- HCM
- Tricuspid regurgitation
- PS

Symptoms

- Small VSDs are common and asymptomatic.
- As pulmonary hypertension develops, fatigue, dyspnoea and symptoms of right ventricular failure.

Pathological considerations

- An isolated VSD is the commonest congenital heart lesion, occurring in 2 per 1,000 births with an equal sex incidence.
- About 50% close spontaneously in infancy.
- As pulmonary vascular resistance falls after delivery there is a left to right shunt.
- Consequent upon the increased flow, irreversible pulmonary changes start in early childhood with initial hypertrophy and secondary thrombotic occlusion of the pulmonary arterioles – leading to pulmonary hypertension.

Investigations

	Very small	Small	Moderate	Large	Eisenmenger's complex
ECG	Normal	Normal	LVH, LAH, LAD	LVH, LAH, RVH	RVH, RAD,
CXR	Normal	Heart normal, mild pulmonary plethora	Slight cardiomegaly, prominent pulmonary arteries and pulmonary plethora	Biventricular enlargement, large pulmonary arteries and plethora	Large pulmonary arteries, no plethora and peripheral pruning

LVH, left ventricular hypertrophy; LAH, left atrial hypertrophy; LAD, left axis deviation
RVH, right ventricular hypertrophy; RAD, right axis deviation.

- Echocardiography and Doppler ultrasonography can show the VSD and can allow the RV pressure to be calculated.
- Magnetic resonance scanning can demonstrate the defect and enable the shunt to be measured.
- Catheterisation confirms the step-up in O_2 saturation in the RV, quantitates the shunt, and diagnoses the site. Aortography will check the valve and exclude PDA or coarctation. RV angiography checks the RV outflow tract.

Management

- All grades need endocarditis prophylaxis.
- Although the surgical morbidity and mortality surrounding correction of small defects is low, surgery is usually unnecessary.
- 30–50% of VSDs close spontaneously, particularly muscular defects and those in the membranous septum. Spontaneous closure does not occur in lesions adjacent to valves or if there is septal malalignment, e.g.:
  - VSD + shift of septum to right – Fallot's tetralogy
  - VSD + shift of septum to left – double-outlet LV with subaortic stenosis.
- Once significant pulmonary resistance has developed, closure of the VSD will be of no benefit.
- Post-MI VSDs require urgent surgery.

7. EISENMENGER'S SYNDROME

Points in the examination

- Centrally cyanosed and plethoric
- Digital clubbing
- Pulse – regular and small volume
- Venous pressure – normal (or raised if RV failure has developed) and the 'a' wave is prominent (the atria are contracting against a raised RV pressure); there may be a prominent 'v' wave (if tricuspid regurgitation)
- Left parasternal heave
- Pulmonary arteries – may be palpable, as may P_2
- There is no thrill (there is insufficient pressure differential to create one)
- S_2 – single and loud (pulmonary hypertension has developed, thus P_2 is loud); there may be a (right ventricular) S_4
- Possible pansystolic murmur over the tricuspid area (TR, if the valve cusp has dilated consequent upon RV failure), as well as an early diastolic murmur over the pulmonary valve (similarly, PA dilatation causing PR – the Graham Steell murmur)

Aetiology

- Cyanotic heart disease in the adult usually occurs in the context of either a congenital VSD, an ASD or PDA.
- As a consequence of the increased pulmonary blood flow, the pulmonary vascular resistance rises.
- When the pulmonary pressure exceeds the systemic pressure the left-to-right shunt reverses to become right to left, and Eisenmenger's syndrome develops.

Differentiating features of the underlying pathologies

- VSD – a single S_2 (equal ventricular pressures)
- ASD – S_2 is widely split and this does not vary with ventilation (A_2 precedes P_2; P_2 does not move, as the increased right ventricular stroke volume does not vary with ventilation)
- PDA – S_2 is normal, i.e. A_2 precedes P_2 and P_2 moves with ventilation; there may be differential cyanosis, pink fingers and blue, clubbed toes (preferential passage of deoxygenated blood into the descending aorta, as the PDA is distal to the origin of the left subclavian artery)

Symptoms

- Failure to thrive, impaired growth, intellectual impairment (if severe)
- Dyspnoea, haemoptysis and frequent chest infections are symptoms of cyanotic heart disease
- Cerebral abscesses, paradoxical emboli, polycythaemia, bleeding diathesis and gout occur

Investigations

- FBC – polycythaemia
- ECG – P pulmonale, RAD, tall R waves, inverted T waves in the right precordial leads (the right ventricular strain pattern), atrial arrhythmias
- CXR – PA dilatation, pruning of the peripheral vessels
- Echo – underlying anatomical defect will be localised, flow seen with Doppler ultrasonography
- Catheter – measures PA pressure and looks for evidence of right-to-left shunting

Management

- Once Eisenmenger's has developed, the mortality rate of heart transplantation negates its use.
- However, heart–lung transplantation offers the only hope of cure for a few young selected patients.
- Give endocarditis prophylaxis.
- Pregnancy should be avoided.
- Perform venesection – to keep the haematocrit below 0.45.

8. PATENT DUCTUS ARTERIOSUS

NB. The ductus arteriosus has to be patent; it is only abnormal if persistent beyond the first month of life. Hence, some prefer the more rational term 'persistent ductus arteriosus'.

Points in the examination

Very small PDA

- May show no signs, save a continuous machinery murmur heard in the 2nd left interspace.
- While there is always a pressure gradient between the aorta and the pulmonary artery, it is greatest towards the end of systole. Thus, while there may be a continuous machinery murmur it is accentuated at about the time of S_2 (which gives the murmur its particular character).
- There may only be a late systolic, or also an early diastolic murmur heard best in expiration at that site, or toward the left clavicle.

In a moderate PDA

- Pulse – full volume and collapsing, regular, rate is normal.
- JVP – normal.
- Apex – displaced inferolaterally and hyperdynamic (the left ventricle is chronically volume-overloaded).
- Thrill – in the second left interspace in systole and/or diastole.
- S_1 normal.
- Continuous machinery murmur in the left 2nd interspace, heard best at the end of systole, in expiration, which may exclude S_2. It radiates towards the left clavicle and may be heard posteriorly.

Aetiology

- It is more common in:
  - Children born prematurely (up to 50%)
  - Females
  - Births at high altitude
  - Maternal rubella infection in the first trimester (PDA is the commonest congenital heart lesion following maternal rubella).

Symptoms

- If small, it is usually picked up routinely or coincidentally in a well, pink, thriving child. CXR and ECG are normal.
- In large shunts they become symptomatic with heart failure.

Differential diagnosis of a continuous murmur

- Pulmonary AV fistulas, coronary AV fistulas, or communications between the ascending aorta and pulmonary artery
- Venous hum – particular care must be taken not to confuse this with the murmur of PDA. Venous hum occurs in young children because of kinking or partial obstruction of one of the larger veins in the neck, thus preventing continuous flow through the vein. It should be suspected because of its loudness in the neck and the youth of the patient! It can be obliterated by pressure on the neck, which completely compresses the offending vein, or merely by altering the position of the neck, or lying flat. Of course, children will not be examined in PACES
- MR and AR
- VSD with AR

Investigations

- ECG – normal or LVH
- CXR – LVH, prominent pulmonary arteries and pulmonary plethora
- Echo and Doppler ultrasonography – demonstrate the shunt
- Catheter with saturation run – to demonstrate other lesions and exclude a VSD

Management

- Infective endocarditis is extremely rare on very small PDAs and these can be left alone.
- Larger PDAs need treating – to avoid failure and endocarditis. Medical therapy is necessary to treat heart failure (which can occur for the first time in adult life).
- Definitive treatment is with ligation or duct occlusion:
  - Many of the problems of ligation have been obviated by the use of duct occluders implanted in patients in the catheter laboratory.
- Irreversible pulmonary hypertension causing Eisenmenger's syndrome is rare, around 5%.

9. TRICUSPID REGURGITATION

Points in the examination

- Pulse – chaotic and of low volume; may rarely be in SR
- Venous pressure – raised, and there are giant systolic 'cv' waves with a rapid 'y' descent, with prominent 'a' waves (only if in SR)
- Left parasternal heave and a soft pansystolic murmur at the left sternal edge, accentuated on inspiration or the Müller manoeuvre (increased venous return to the right side)
- S_3 – may be heard at the left sternal edge
- One must proceed to examine the lungs for a cause of pulmonary hypertension, as well as the abdomen and beyond, for the peripheral signs of tricuspid regurgitation:
  - Peripheral and central cyanosis
  - Ascites and other signs of chronic liver disease
  - Tender pulsatile hepatomegaly
  - Peripheral oedema

Aetiology

- Functional – commonest:
  - Secondary to pulmonary hypertension.
- Organic – uncommon:
  - Infective endocarditis – IV drug abusers
  - Floppy tricuspid valve (TV) may be associated with the floppy mitral valve (MV) associated with congenital heart disease, either as a primary phenomenon (e.g. tricuspid atresia/hypoplasia and Ebstein's anomaly) or secondary to right heart enlargement (e.g. ASD)
  - Rheumatic tricuspid valve disease invariably occurs in association with aortic and mitral valve disease
  - Rarer causes are tricuspid endocarditis as part of the carcinoid syndrome, and secondary to the centrally acting appetite suppressants phentermine, fenfluramine and dexfenfluramine (all of which have been withdrawn because of reports of the development of valvular disease).
- NB. In establishing the diagnosis of tricuspid regurgitation, the presence of a systolic murmur is of less importance than the observation of a giant systolic 'cv' wave followed by a rapid 'y' descent in the JVP.

Symptoms

- Abdominal distension and discomfort
- Hepatic angina
- Jaundice
- Peripheral oedema
- Fatigue and dyspnoea

Investigations

- ECG – AF, P pulmonale (if in SR), RV hypertrophy
- Echo – dilated or hypertrophic RV, functional TV disease, vegetations, magnitude of regurgitant jet on Doppler ultrasonography
- Cardiac catheter

Management

- Management of the underlying lung disease
- Diuretics
- Fluid restriction
- Surgery
- Annuloplasty or plication
- Valve replacement (rarely)

10. HYPERTROPHIC OBSTRUCTIVE CARDIOMYOPATHY

Points in the examination

- Pulse – normal volume, may be jerky in character with a large tidal wave.
- Apex – prominent, minimally displaced, pressure-loaded apical impulse with a characteristic lift. The atrial impulse can often be felt – the double apex. The LV can be described as muscular.
- Systolic thrill – present at the lower left sternal edge.
- Apical S_4; S_2 is reversed in severe HCM.
- A harsh ejection systolic murmur (ESM) starts well after S_1, radiates from the apex to the LSE and towards the axilla. The murmur is accentuated by forced expiration or the Valsalva manoeuvre (raising the intrathoracic pressure), and is diminished by deep inspiration or the Müller manoeuvre.
- May hear a mid-diastolic rumble in inflow obstruction.
- The systolic murmur of HCM can radiate to the apex and axilla. It can also merge with the mitral regurgitation caused by the systolic anterior motion (SAM) of the anterior mitral valve leaflet.

Aetiology

- Up to 70% of cases are inherited as an autosomal dominant condition with a variable degree of penetrance and equal sex distribution. Spontaneous mutations occur and account for the rest.
- There is a large degree of genetic heterogeneity which accounts for the wide clinical spectrum of HCM, e.g. there are over 30 missense mutations in the cardiac β-myosin heavy chain on chromosome 14, which account for a third of cases.
- Mutations on the gene coding for troponin-T at 1q3 carry the worst prognosis.
- The identification of the gene in an individual or family may enable an earlier and more precise diagnosis, and enable more useful prognostic information to be given.
- The pathogenesis is unknown, but the microscopic features of thickened and haphazardly arranged muscle fibres may be the result of excessive catecholamine stimulation due to a genetic abnormality of neural crest tissue. (NB. Association between HCM, hypertension, lentiginosis and phaeochromocytoma)

Differential diagnosis

- Aortic stenosis:
  - The pulse in AS is slow-rising not jerky, the thrill is at the base, there is often an ejection sound and manoeuvres to vary obstruction do not change the murmur.
- Subvalvar mitral regurgitation, e.g. chordal rupture.
- VSD:
  - In VSD and subvalvar MR the pulse can be jerky, the thrill anterior or at the left sternal edge with a late or ESM. Therefore the key feature to look for is the lack of variability with manoeuvres to vary the obstruction, e.g. Müller and Valsalva manoeuvres.

Symptoms

- It is often asymptomatic.
- Can present at any age with palpitations (associated with Wolff–Parkinson–White (WPW) syndrome), syncope or sudden death as in AS.
- Angina can occur even with normal coronary arteries.
- Dyspnoea can be due to a stiff left ventricle in diastole, thus reducing atrial transport.

Symptoms may become rapidly worse if AF develops. Mitral regurgitation often coexists.

Investigations

- CXR – often normal unless heart failure has developed.
- ECG – usually non-specifically abnormal even in asymptomatic patients:
  - LVH plus ST- and T-wave changes, progressive and steeper T-wave inversion with time
  - Q waves in inferior and lateral leads – septal hypertrophy and fibrosis
  - Pre-excitation and WPW syndrome
  - Ventricular ectopics
  - Exercise ECG – maximum oxygen ventilation capacity is reduced; 1 in 3 patients have a fall in blood pressure; 1 in 4 get ST changes
  - 24-h ECG – ventricular tachycardia.
- Echocardiography – several features in association are diagnostic:
  - Mid-systolic aortic valve closure
  - Asymmetrical septal hypertrophy
  - Small LV cavity with a hypercontractile posterior wall
  - Systolic anterior motion (SAM) of the mitral valve.

- Catheter – echocardiography has reduced the need to pass a catheter into the excitable and unstable LV, which often induces VT. But it does document the withdrawal gradient, any MR and the coronary arteries; it is also used for electrophysiological studies in the WPW syndrome.

Management

- Nitrates should be avoided for angina as they increase the outflow obstruction (thus a useful diagnostic test with amyl nitrate).
- β-Blockers are the mainstay of treatment for giddiness, syncope, angina, dyspnoea.
- Amiodarone is given for SVT.
- Infective endocarditis may occur.
- Although it is well tolerated in pregnancy, there is a strong possibility the child will be affected.
- Genetic testing, but the genotype–phenotype correlation is currently uncertain.
- Dual-chamber pacing with depolarisation from the RV apex alters septal motion and is a promising alternative to surgery. Dual-chamber pacing is required as atrial transport is so important in HCM.
- Surgical myotomy or myomectomy through the aortic valve effectively reduces the left ventricular outflow tract gradient more than pacing but with a higher mortality risk.

11. PROSTHETIC VALVE

Points in the examination

- The abnormal heart sound is the prosthetic valve. There may be an opening sound.
- Look for the distal stigmata of infective endocarditis, particularly fever, splenomegaly, haematuria and splinter haemorrhages.
- A forward-flow murmur, e.g. ESM across an aortic valve or diastolic murmur over an MV, is normal. They are particularly prominent with mechanical valves.
- A regurgitant murmur, e.g. a systolic murmur across an MV, should always be regarded as pathological and indicative of valve failure.
- Look for evidence of valve failure:
  - Regurgitation and heart failure.
- Inspect the teeth – meticulous dental care is vital.
- The opening and closing sounds of either ball or disc should be clear and sharp and not muffled. Vegetations may muffle the sounds and restrict movement.
- Are there stigmata of anticoagulation or embolic disease?

Aetiology

Mechanical valves

- Ball-and-cage – Starr–Edwards: the mitral valve has four struts, while the aortic valve has three; the silastic ball is invisible on X-ray.
- Single- and double-tilting discs:
  - All require anticoagulation for life
  - More durable, but greater risk of thromboembolism than xenografts
  - The partner can be disturbed by the audible clicks.

Biological valves

- Xenografts – either porcine valves or pericardium mounted on a frame; only the frame is visible:
  - Patients with aortic valves do not require anticoagulation; however, most prosthetic mitral valves are inserted in patients with AF, who thus require anticoagulation
  - They are less durable and need replacing in 8–10 years
  - They are less durable in younger patients, but better in the elderly.
- Homografts – cadaveric aortic or pulmonary valves. They are the first choice in a young patient needing an aortic valve, but they may degrade with time.

Symptoms

- Prosthetic valve endocarditis:
  - Any unexplained malaise, fever, weight loss, dyspnoea, etc.; patients will be told to avoid antibiotics until seen by a cardiologist
  - Any dental treatment in the last 6 months with no antibiotics
  - Change in valve sounds
  - New symptoms, however vague.
- Systemic embolisation:
  - Commonest with mechanical valves, approximately 1% per year even with ideal anticoagulation.
- Dyspnoea, associated with a failing valve – this is a predictable feature of biological valves which fail more rapidly than mechanical valves.
- Haemolysis, valve thrombosis, valve dehiscence, myocardial failure and arrhythmias occur.

Investigations and management

- CXR.
- If endocarditis occurs on a prosthetic valve it results in a mortality of up to 60%. The patient requires urgent referral to a cardiothoracic centre. Most cases require a valve replacement, after prolonged systemic antibiotics.
- If systemic embolisation occurs check for endocarditis:
  - Cultures
  - FBC, ESR and CRP
  - Echo – vegetations or intracardiac thrombi, as well as ensuring adequacy of anticoagulation
  - 24-h tape – consider transient arrhythmias
  - Dipyridamole and aspirin may need to be added, or the valve may need replacing.

- Pregnancy – historically women of childbearing age received bioprostheses due to theoretical concerns of fetal abnormalities with warfarin.

The Neurological Examination

1: General

When considering the neurological system there are a few points to note:
- A full neurological examination may take the best part of a day. In PACES, time is limited to 10 minutes, and thus one must direct the examination to some degree.
- The examination serves three purposes:
  - Where is the pathology?
  - What is it?
  - To screen the other areas of the nervous system for disease.
- In PACES, although the instructions given outside the room will direct the examination, other areas that may be of interest must still be considered.
- You are likely to be asked to examine one of the following:
  - The upper limbs
  - The lower limbs
  - Cranial nerves.
- You can also be asked to examine the:
  - Cerebellar system
  - Motor or sensory system
  - Speech
  - Eyes.
- The following may need to be included in examination:
  - The spine and skull for injury or disease
  - Cranial bruits around the orbit, or elsewhere as necessary
  - Carotid artery bruits.

GENERAL EXAMINATION

- Appropriate dress and appearance of the patient?
- Strength of the patient's handshake, as appropriate.
- As you introduce yourself, consider whether:
  - Is what they say appropriate? It is a good idea to ask a couple of questions surreptitiously: 'Good morning, I am Dr...., could you tell me your name please?'; 'Are you right- or left-handed?'

(This question should be asked unless the information is given.); and 'Are you quite comfortable?'
- Is there dysarthria or dysphonia? (Formal examination of speech is dealt with later.)
- Is there any reason to suggest a disorder of higher mental function or thought process? A mental state assessment is not necessary, unless specifically requested.

GENERAL INSPECTION

Look for:
- Asymmetry:
  - Poverty of movement
  - Wasting or hypertrophy
  - Fasciculation
  - Posture of limbs
  - Abnormal movements
  - Injuries – burns, cuts, ulcers or deformed joints
  - Signs of systemic disease – diabetes, acromegaly, Paget's disease or hydrocephalus

CRANIAL NERVES

- Position the patient so they are sitting over the edge of a bed if possible.
- Look carefully at the face for ptosis, proptosis, asymmetry, the scalp and eyebrows for craniotomy scars, the skin for neurofibromas or naevi (e.g. Sturge–Weber syndrome).

Olfactory

- Not tested routinely. However, if it is required, bottles of standard smells should be provided and held under each nostril in turn. Anosmia is most commonly bilateral – upper respiratory infection, meningioma of the olfactory groove, ethmoid tumours, basal or frontal skull fracture, after pituitary surgery, congenital (e.g. Kallman's syndrome), smoking and increasing age. Unilateral – head trauma, early olfactory groove meningiomas.

Ophthalmic

- Look at the eyes.
- Assess acuity, fields and fundi.
- Acuity – with the patient wearing their normal spectacles, or using a pinhole (refractive errors are not considered abnormalities of the cranial nerves), test each eye in turn with a Snellen chart, ideally placed on a wall 6 m away from the patient:
  - Normal acuity is 6/6. If less than this, the lower number is the line they can read. If the patient cannot read the top line. i.e. 6/60, move closer; if they cannot read it at 1 m, i.e. 1/60, ask them to count fingers at 1 m. Failing this, perception of hand movements at 30 cm, then light acuity, is tested
  - Although any lesion from the cornea, aqueous, lens, vitreous, fundus, or optic nerve pathway can cause reduced acuity, in the neurological examination it is usually due to nerve or pathway pathology
  - Bilateral sudden blindness – bilateral occipital lobe infarction or trauma; bilateral optic nerve damage, e.g. methyl alcohol damage, and hysteria
  - Unilateral sudden blindness – retinal artery emboli, retinal vein thrombosis, retinal detachment, temporal arteritis, occasionally optic neuritis and migraine
  - Unilateral/bilateral gradual blindness – cataracts, glaucoma, macular degeneration, diabetic retinopathy, optic nerve or chiasmal compression, nerve damage, e.g. tobacco amblyopia.
- Fields are examined by confronting the patient (without their glasses) with a red-topped hat-pin:
  - You must be at the same level as the patient with the pin held equidistant between you and the patient. The patient must cover the eye not under test with the palm (scrunching the eye is unacceptable) and look into your eye. Make sure they can see the pin, and that it is red when held centrally. Move the pin slowly inwards from your periphery; the point of initial vision marks out the patient's periphery and when it becomes red this indicates central vision. Repeat the procedure in each quadrant of each eye. The pin head disappears at the blind spot, which is enlarged in neuritis and papilloedema. Scotomas are peripheral defects within the field, seen in neuritis and occasionally chiasmal compression. The use of moving fingers is insensitive and should only be used for screening.
- Also test for sensory inattention in the fields. (Sensory inattention – in sensory lesions above the thalamus, the first detectable sign is inattention. Sensation can appear normal when both sides are tested

individually; however, when tested simultaneously, the abnormal cortex will ignore the stimulus. Thus with a right-sided lesion, the patient will ignore the stimulus on the left.)
- Fundoscopy (see examination of the eyes, p. 383).

Oculomotor, trochlear and abducens

- Test pupillary reflexes, accommodation and eye movements.
- In good light with the patient looking into the distance, note pupil size, shape, equality and regularity; look for ptosis (bilateral ptosis is easy to miss).
- Light reflex – the patient must look into the distance so they do not accommodate; do not shine the light at the fovea as it is painful. Look for the direct and consensual reflexes on both sides; both should be equally brisk.
- To test for a relative afferent pupillary defect or Marcus Gunn pupil, employ the swinging light test. Move the torch in an arc from pupil to pupil. If there is optic atrophy, neuritis or reduced acuity, the affected pupil will dilate (rather than constrict) when the torch is moved from the normal to the abnormal eye. (Shining the light in the healthy eye causes rapid constriction to both eyes. Subsequently, when the light is moved to the affected eye the impaired afferent limb results in slow transmission, allowing time for the pupils to dilate.)
- Accommodation – place your finger about 30 cm in front of the patient's eyes and ask them to look into the distance, and then to focus onto your finger. The eyes should adduct, intort and the pupils should constrict. Intact accommodation with an absent light reflex occurs in patients with diabetes mellitus and neurosyphilis – the Argyll Robertson pupil where the pupils are small and irregular, and the Holmes–Adie pupil where it is larger, regular and reacts sluggishly to accommodation.
- There are six cardinal directions of gaze. The patient should be asked if they see double in a particular place; if the images are side by side, then only the lateral or medial recti can be responsible. Separation is greatest in the direction of movement of the affected muscle, or the direction in which the weak muscle has its purest action. Move your finger like a letter H, thus allowing the action of each muscle to be assessed. If diplopia is present at maximum separation of the object, cover the eyes in turn. When the outer image is lost this is the eye and thus the muscle involved. If diplopia persists with one eye covered it may be lens dislocation, astigmatism or factitious. If the pattern of loss is complex and cannot easily be explained, always consider Graves' disease or myasthenia.

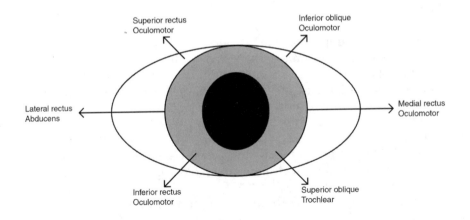

- Is there internuclear ophthalmoplegia? Failure of adduction of one eye, when the contralateral is abducted (e.g. on attempted gaze to the left, the left eye abducts normally but the right eye fails to adduct. As the left eye abducts you know that the mechanism down to and including the pontine centre for lateral gaze (adjacent to the VIth nucleus) is intact. As convergence is normal one knows that the IIIrd nucleus and medial rectus are intact. Thus the lesion lies between the two in the medial longitudinal fascicle (MLF) on the same side as the adducting eye). It is closely allied to ataxic nystagmus, where the abducting eye, having crossed the midline, goes into a fine, quick, well-sustained nystagmus; the contralateral eye fails to pass the mid-position.
- These signs have immense bearing on examination of the eyes:
    - First, when testing gaze, if the object is held too close then a convergent gaze will conceal an internuclear ophthalmoplegia
    - Second, the above signs aid localisation – an internuclear ophthalmoplegia (INO) with a contralateral hemiparesis is indicative of brainstem disease
    - Last, a gradual onset of an INO which is usually bilateral is highly suggestive of MS. A sudden onset with facial numbness is more in keeping with stroke.
- Hold lateral gaze to check for nystagmus, remembering that at extremes of gaze nystagmus (see p. 265) becomes physiological; and upwards for fatiguability – ptosis (see p. 263) may appear.

Trigeminal

- The territory supplied by the Vth nerve is often well illustrated in Sturge–Weber syndrome or herpes zoster. It covers the anterior two-thirds of the crown but does not supply the angle of the jaw. People with simulated disease are unlikely to have impaired sensation over the scalp but normal sensation over the angle of the jaw.
- Inspect for wasting of the temporalis and masseter muscles. Loss of bulk is best appreciated on palpation while the patient clenches their teeth. On opening the mouth the jaw will be deviate to the affected side, pushed by the intact lateral pterygoids. The motor root runs with the mandibular division.
- The jaw jerk is normally absent or just present. It is prominent in an upper motor neurone (UMN) lesion, e.g. pseudobulbar palsy
- Test sensation in each division: ophthalmic, maxillary and mandibular. Look for sensory inattention. The mandibular division is not involved in cavernous sinus disease as Vc has already left the skull through the foramen ovale.
- Elicit the corneal reflex, touch but do not wipe the cornea, nor test the conjunctiva. The patient blinks, as the efferent limb is the VIIth nerve. Loss may be the first sign of pathology, e.g. in acoustic neuroma. When herpes zoster damages the nerve, corneal involvement is more likely if the nasociliary branch on the side of the nose is also affected. Never test over the central part of the cornea, as in corneal anaesthesia to do so would risk corneal ulceration and subsequent visual impairment.

Facial

- Inspect for asymmetry; symmetry is retained in bilateral disease.
- In theory it is easy to distinguish between UMN and lower motor neurone (LMN) lesions as the latter affect the whole face. The sparing of the upper part of the face in UMN pyramidal lesions reflects its bilateral cortical innervation. The involuntary movements of the face, such as smiling and frowning, are subcortical, bilaterally represented and therefore little, if at all, affected in UMN pyramidal lesions.
  - Ask the patient to close their eyes; try to push against the corrugations on the forehead or open the eye. Are the eyelashes equally buried? Bell's phenomenon may be seen, where the eyeballs are seen to rotate upwards on closing the eyes. Although present in everyone, it is only visible with weakness of the orbicularis oculi in LMN lesions. The nasolabial fold is smoothed.

- While attempting to smile, or show their teeth, the patient's mouth is drawn to the normal side.
- They cannot whistle.
- Ask them to inflate their cheeks, and tap on each side. Air can be made to escape more easily on the affected side.
- Involvement of platysma is demonstrated on attempted eversion of the bottom lip.
- It is unlikely that you will be required to test taste on the anterior two-thirds of the patient's tongue[2]. The practical importance is that loss of taste indicates a lesion proximal to the point where the chorda tympani joins the facial nerve and is a poor prognostic sign.
- Hyperacusis may occur if the nerve to the stapedius is affected, i.e. lesions proximal to the stylomastoid foramen.
- Check the external auditory meatus for herpes zoster lesions in association with a LMN VIIth nerve palsy – Ramsay Hunt syndrome. The geniculate ganglion is not always involved and the weakness probably reflects direct invasion of the facial nerve.
- Unilateral LMN weakness is usually due to damage in the temporal bone, e.g. Bell's palsy, zoster, trauma or infections, or beyond the stylomastoid foramen in Bell's palsy or trauma, accident or carcinoma of the parotid glands. Bilateral weakness is often due to myasthenia, dystrophia myotonica, sarcoidosis or facioscapulohumeral dystrophy or, rarely, acute infective polyneuritis – Miller Fisher variant of Guillain–Barré syndrome. In all these conditions, the levator palpebrae superioris is also affected so that ptosis is present. Bilateral weakness of the facial nerve is very difficult to recognise; a clue may be an expressionless face.

Vestibulocochlear

- Inspect the external auditory meatus and the drum with an otoscope if disease expected.
- Test gross hearing by whispering '68' or '77' (high tones) and '100' or '22' (low tones), 30 cm from the patient's ear, at the end of expiration, while moving your fingers against the other ear.

---

2 For testing taste, use strong solutions of common salt and sugar and weak solutions of citric acid and quinine for 'salt', 'sweet', 'sour' and 'bitter', respectively. Apply the solutions with a wooden rod on either side of the tongue, then ask the patient to indicate sensation by pointing to a card before putting their tongue back into their mouth, as this can reflect taste on the posterior one-third (glossopharyngeal nerve). Ask the patient to rinse their mouth between tastes. Use quinine last.

- Using a 256-Hz tuning fork ideally, perform Rinné's and Weber's tests. Rinné's test is normal/positive when air conduction is greater than bone; if abnormal/negative there is conductive deafness. Weber's test, when the fork is placed in the middle of the forehead, will localise to the normal nerve in nerve deafness or towards the abnormal ear in conductive deafness.
- If vertigo is mentioned in the scenario, perform Hallpike's manoeuvre. Tell the patient what you are about to do. Have them sit up and then quickly drop them back so their head is 30° below horizontal, turned 30° toward the examiner with their eyes open looking at the ceiling. If positive, after a short pause there will be vertigo and nystagmus to the lower ear for up to a minute. It is not reproducible for 10–15 minutes and indicates benign positional vertigo. If it occurs immediately and is not fatiguable it indicates a central cause, e.g. brainstem disease.
- Acoustic neurofibromas present insidiously with unilateral deafness, followed by ataxia and headache. Tinnitus is common but patients rarely complain of vertigo. The corneal reflex is lost first, then papilloedema, nystagmus and signs of an ipsilateral cerebellar lesion occur if large. The nearby VIth and VIIth nerves can be affected.

Glossopharyngeal and vagus

- Inspect the palate with a torch; is the uvula central?
- Ask them to say 'Ah'. If there is unilateral weakness of the Xth nerve the uvula will move to the normal side.
- Check the gag reflex – sensory IXth nerve and motor limb Xth nerve. Thus if sensation is intact but contraction is absent this suggests a X-nerve lesion – the most common cause of a reduced gag is old age.
- Ask them to speak and cough – recurrent laryngeal nerves.
- The gag has no bearing on swallowing ability, but gives an indication of the ability to protect the airway. Swallowing should be tested separately with a glass of water, if necessary.
- Taste is not routinely assessed.
- Isolated glossopharyngeal lesions are very rare.
- In both bulbar and pseudobulbar palsy the voice is nasal. In both, the palate fails to move when the patient says 'Ah'. However, the gag in pseudobulbar palsy is exaggerated, as it is an UMN lesion, whereas it is absent in bulbar palsy.

Accessory

- Ask the patient to shrug their shoulders, which tests the trapezius, and turn their head to the side for the sternomastoids. Feel the muscles.
- Damage is usually due to inflammation or operation on the upper cervical lymph nodes. It has also been reported in a doctor whose neck was 'bitten vigorously by a nurse in the course of an obviously friendly love-making session'!

Hypoglossal

- Inspect the tongue in the mouth. The XII nerve is purely motor; in UMN lesions (e.g. pseudobulbar palsy) the tongue is small and immobile, in LMN lesions (e.g. bulbar palsy) it is wasted and fasciculates.
- Ask them to protrude their tongue; it will deviate to the weak side in unilateral disease.
- Isolated disease is rare.
- In the jugular foramen syndrome, because the IX, X and XI (XII exits close by in the hypoglossal foramen) nerves all leave the skull together, damage affects them all. The syndrome is more common than isolated lesions. It can occur in nasopharyngeal carcinoma, trauma, Paget's disease, meningitis, basilar aneurysms and the rare glomus jugulare tumour.

2: Peripheral Nervous System

OBSERVATION AND INSPECTION

- Look generally around the bed (e.g. wheelchair, walking stick, shoes – callipers, built-up heels, scuffed toes).
- Ensure the patient is adequately exposed before considering the following points.
- Posture – disease of the pyramidal tracts gives a classic appearance. There is increased resistance to passive movement, which is more marked in the flexors of the upper and the extensors of the lower limb. Thus, the upper limb is held adducted, flexed at the elbow, wrist and finger and pronated at the forearm, while the lower limb, being held in extension, can still act as a useful prop.
- Bulk – wasting can signify denervated muscle, primary muscle disease or disuse atrophy, e.g. because of pain. Look at the pattern: is it proximal, distal or generalised, symmetrical or asymmetrical (e.g. poliomyelitis)?
- Abnormal movements:
  - Fasciculation – seen in motor neurone disease (MND) (LMN involvement), motor root compression and peripheral neuropathy. In the absence of other signs of disease it is usually benign – the rule to follow is that it is only significant in the presence of muscle weakness, wasting and reflex changes. Do not tap the muscles to induce it, as fasciculation is the *spontaneous* discharge of individual motor units.
  - Tremor – this is a rhythmical involuntary movement of any part of the body, commonly the hands. Decide which parts of the body are tremulous, pay particular attention to the lips, tongue, chin, head and limbs. Look for any features of Parkinson's syndrome. The main categories are resting, postural and intention:
    - resting tremor – characteristic of Parkinson's syndrome (see p. 247), in which it is coarse ('pill rolling') and often worse on one side
    - postural
    - physiological – fine tremor, equally present in both hands; enhanced in thyrotoxicosis, anxiety and by adrenergic drugs or caffeine
    - essential – coarse tremor, often worse in one hand. It is important to differentiate this from a parkinsonian tremor. Examine the patient's gait, look at the face, listen to the voice; do they gesticulate when talking freely?

- intention – cerebellar disease (see p. 244). This tremor only appears as the hand approaches the target. Look for confirmatory signs of cerebellar disease
- NB. A coarse, proximal ('bat wing') tremor in a young patient should alert you to the rare possibility of Wilson's disease.
- Spontaneous movements:
  - orofacial or tardive dyskinesia (e.g. neuroleptic drugs; Parkinson's – 'dopa-induced dyskinesia'
  - tics
  - chorea – Huntington's
  - myoclonus
  - dystonia.
- Skin – neurofibroma, herpes zoster, purpura (glucocorticosteroids), rashes, lipohypertrophy.
- Shake hands – myotonia, wasting of the small muscles, see later.

LOWER LIMBS

Gait

- If asked to examine the lower limbs, first ask the patient to walk several metres, turn and walk back. It may need repeating in difficult cases. If afraid they may fall, ask a nurse or the examiner to assist the patient; gait cannot otherwise be examined.
- Make a note of stride length, arm swinging, posture, base and involuntary movements.
- Have the patient stand on their toes, a sensitive test for weakness of gastrocnemius and soleus muscles.
- Ask the patient to stand on their heels, failure to do so demonstrates foot drop:
  - Unilateral foot drop – one leg lifted higher than the other and the foot hangs down while elevated; usually a common peroneal lesion
  - Bilateral foot drop – bilateral high steppage gait with the feet slapping the ground when they hit; often caused by a peripheral neuropathy, e.g. hereditary motor sensory neuropathy (HMSN) -1 and -2.
- A similar steppage gait is seen in sensory ataxia, but the base is broad and patients watch the floor intently. Perform Romberg's test (see p. 214).

- Hemiplegic – one leg is held stiffly and circumducts on walking, the foot is inverted and the toes scrape the floor (look at the shoes); the arm is held stiffly, flexed at the side.
- Spastic paraplegic gait – both legs are held stiffly and circumduct, the feet are inverted and may cross (scissor). The florid form is seen in longstanding spastic paraparesis, e.g. cerebral palsy or hereditary spastic paraplegia.
- Parkinsonian – small steps, little arm swinging, stooped posture, festination, turning is laborious and freezing may occur. In early disease one arm failing to swing may be the only feature.
- *Marche petit pas* (walk with a small step) – very similar to parkinsonian gait, but broad-based and they are upright. Seen in normal-pressure hydrocephalus and multilacunar infarcts (dementia, pseudobulbar palsy, emotional lability).
- Cerebellar – broad-based, irregular, tendency to veer to one side or the other, staggering on turning. To see if the patient consistently falls to one side ask the patient to march on the spot with eyes open and closed, walk heel to toe or round a chair. Patients with vermal lesions may stagger in any direction; on sitting they may wobble.
- Antalgic – the good limb hurries through and the painful limb buckles to cushion the impact on each stride.
- If patients have an abnormal gait but no weakness, spasticity, rigidity, akinesia, sensory loss or ataxia they probably have a truncal ataxia due to a midline cerebellar lesion, most commonly secondary to alcohol. Another consideration is dyspraxia due to a frontal lobe lesion.
- Romberg's test – have the patient stand between you and a wall (in case they fall). If they are large and you fear the test may be positive, ask for assistance. Romberg noted that patients with tabes dorsalis (loss of dorsal columns) could not stand with their feet together and eyes closed. An increase in body sway on closing the eyes is not a positive Romberg's test as it can occur in other causes of poor balance. The term 'positive Rombergism' is best reserved for those patients who would fall if they closed their eyes.
- Pes cavus – a high arch with clawing of the toes in a 'thick' foot, e.g. HMSN, Friedreich's ataxia and spina bifida.

Tone

- Palpate the thighs, hamstrings and calves; this is essential to assess tone effectively, especially if it is reduced.
- Roll the lower limb from side to side before suddenly lifting the knee; the foot should not leave the bed:
  - UMN lesions – the tone is spastic and clasp-knife
  - LMN lesions – flaccid paralysis, decreased tone, look for fasciculations again (expect reduced reflexes)
  - Extrapyramidal disease – 'lead pipe' rigidity where the resistance is present throughout the range of movement; if tremor is superimposed then 'cogwheel' rigidity is felt
  - Cerebellar disease – hypotonia.
- Test for ankle (knee bent, thigh externally rotated, maintain dorsiflexion) and knee clonus.

Power

- It is customary to grade power on a 5–0 scale:
  - 5 – normal power
  - 4 – movement against gravity and resistance
  - 3 – active movement against gravity
  - 2 – active movement, with gravity eliminated
  - 1 – flicker or trace of contraction
  - 0 – no contraction
- However, subdivision of grade 4 is helpful, thus:
  - 4 –, 4 and 4+ indicate movement against slight, moderate and strong resistance, respectively. Grade 4 power is never normal and warrants an explanation
  - The movements to be tested are shown in the table below, along with their muscle, nerve and root innervation; the dominant root is shown in bold:

Action	Muscle	Nerve	Segmental level
Hip flexion	Iliopsoas	Femoral	**L1, L2**, L3
Hip extension	Gluteus maximus	Inferior gluteal	**L5, S1**, S2
Hip adduction	Adductors	Obturator	**L2, L3**, L4
Knee flexion	Hamstrings	Sciatic	L5, **S1**, S2
Knee extension	Quadriceps	Femoral	L2, **L3, L4**
Ankle dorsiflexion	Tibialis anterior	Deep peroneal	**L4**, L5
Ankle plantarflexion	Gastrocnemius	Tibial	S1, S2
Ankle inversion	Tibialis posterior	Tibial	L5, **S1, S2**
Ankle eversion	Peroneus longus and brevis	Superficial peroneal	L5, S1

Reflexes

- Short-handled reflex hammers should not be used in PACES. Strike the tendon reflexes firmly, once.
- They can be pathologically brisk in UMN lesions (+++), or brisk (++) in anxious or young slender people. They are absent (–) or present only on reinforcement (±) in LMN lesions, although loss of the ankle jerk is common in those over 70 years of age. You must check for reinforcement (e.g. Jendrassik manoeuvre) if a reflex is absent. Compare the sides.
- Ankle – S1:
  - This reflex is of key importance, so relax and put the patient at ease. This may be easier to elicit on the sole of the foot, or even with them kneeling on a chair with slight dorsiflexion applied. If it is absent, actively consider cauda equina pathology as it is extremely easy to miss in a 'routine' neurological examination. Is plantar flexion normal? Is there a catheter? Make sure you examine the sacral sensation on the back of the limb and mention you would like to examine sensation over the buttock and perineum and assess anal tone. To fail to do so is a serious error. Analogous to spinal cord compression, if the compression is not noticed and relieved promptly, permanent sphincter damage can occur. With consequent renal damage this can be fatal.
- Knee – L2, L3, L4.
- Plantar – corticospinal tract (afferent L5, S1):
  - Gently scratch a key or a stick along the outer edge of the sole of the foot towards the little toe, then medially along the metatarsus. This causes contraction of the tensor fascia lata, often with contraction of the adductors and sartorius. As the stimulus increases, flexion of the toes occurs, from lateral to medial, at the metatarsus. The ankle dorsiflexes and inverts. It is never completely absent in normal individuals. Scratching medially can induce a grasp reflex which is a different sign, see below.
    - an extensor response (Babinski's sign) is only found in corticospinal tract lesions and is thus pathognomic of UMN pathology. In major corticospinal lesions the area from which an extensor response can be elicited (receptive field) enlarges, such that Oppenheim's sign (pressing on the medial border of the tibia) becomes positive.

Coordination

- Heel–shin test – ask the patient, with their eyes open, to elevate the lower limb straight in the air, then place the heel on the knee and run it straight down the shin, then repeat. Compare the sides.
- Proximal weakness – ask the patient to make circles with the foot at the ankle.
- Dysdiadochokinesis – ask the patient to tap a foot repeatedly on your palm.
- Truncal ataxia – the limbs are often completely normal in lesions of the vermis, but on asking the patient to sit up with their arms folded they usually sway from side to side, or fall over. They may have difficulty standing, and their gait is characteristic.

Sensation

- Test the sensation in the dermatomes L1 (inguino/femoral region), L2 (lateral thigh), L3 (knee and medial thigh), L4 (medial calf), L5 (lateral calf down to the great toe), S1 (lateral foot, sole and heel) and S2 (back of knee and thigh). Compare left and right.
- There is considerable overlap of dermatomes and thus an isolated root lesion, e.g. L5 caused by a disc prolapse at L4/5, may only cause a patch of sensory loss, in this case on the dorsum of the foot.
- Test from abnormal to normal, having first demonstrated to the patient what normal feels like, usually on the anterior chest.
    - NB. The dorsal columns decussate in the medulla, while pain and temperature fibres enter the cord before crossing a few segments higher to ascend in the spinothalamic tract.
    - Light touch (dorsal columns and spinothalamic tracts) – dab the patient with a wisp of cotton wool. Never stroke the cotton wool as this stimulates the spinothalamic tract.
    - Vibration sense (dorsal columns) – using a 128-Hz tuning fork at the great toe, move proximally to the medial malleolus, knee, iliac crest and sternum as necessary. If the patient detects the feeling of vibration ask them to say when it stops before deadening the fork with your fingers. Individuals can usually detect vibration for more than 10 seconds; it is useful in quantifying progressive impairment.
    - Proprioception (dorsal columns) – first explain to the patient what are up and down. Grip the toe by the sides so as not to stimulate pressure sensation. Normally a few degrees of movement is detected. Move proximally as necessary.

- Pain (spinothalamic tracts) – only when you have gained the patient's confidence is it prudent to test pain; use a clean neurological pin, never a hat-pin. Ask them to say when it feels normal or if a pin feels sharp or blunt. Is there dissociated sensory loss, e.g. syringomyelia?
- Temperature (spinothalamic tracts) can be tested if necessary, with test tubes of warm and cold water.
- If a stocking sensory loss is present, demonstrate that the sensory loss is present right round the limb.
- If compression of the cord is suspected, then demonstrate a sensory level. This is often asymmetric.

UPPER LIMBS

Drift

- Look at the outstretched upper limbs for drift – the patient's palms facing upwards and with eyes closed:
  - UMN lesions – the hand falls and the forearm pronates, the movement starts distally and moves proximally
  - Cerebellar disease – the arms drift upwards
  - Sensory ataxia – with decreased joint position sense, the fingers display pseudoathetosis, 'Romberg's sign', in the fingers.

Tone

- Roll the wrist and flex and extend the elbow in a random manner. Feel the muscles.
- Greater resistance to passive movement occurs in the pronators compared to the supinators in the forearm in early UMN lesions.

Power

- The movements to be tested are shown in the table opposite, along with their muscle, nerve and root innervation; the dominant root is in bold. Graded 1–5, as in the legs:

Action	Muscle	Nerve	Segmental level
Shoulder abduction	Deltoid	Axillary	**C5**, C6
Elbow flexion	Biceps	Musculo-cutaneous	C5, C6
Elbow extension	Triceps	Radial	C6, **C7**, C8
Wrist extension	Extensor carpi ulnaris and radialis	Radial	C5, **C6**, C7, **C8**
Wrist flexion, and abduction	Flexor carpi radialis	Median	C6, C7
Wrist flexion, and adduction	Flexor carpi ulnaris	Ulnar	C7, **C8**, T1
Finger extension	Extensor digitorum	Radial	C7, C8
Opposition of thumb	Opponens pollicis	Median	C8, **T1**
Abduction of thumb	Abductor pollicis brevis	Median	C8, **T1**
Abduction of the index finger	1st dorsal interosseous	Ulnar	C8, **T1**
Adduction of the index finger	2nd palmar interosseous	Ulnar	C8, **T1**

Reflexes

- Biceps – C5, C6.
- Supinator – C6, C7.
- Triceps – C7, C8.
- Grade as before, with reinforcement, if necessary.
- In addition, a number of other reflexes can be elicited:
  - Abdominal reflex – gently scratching towards the umbilicus in the four quadrants of the stomach causes reflex contraction of the recti in normal individuals. They are commonly lost with age, obesity or after abdominal surgery. However, it is a curious feature of UMN pathology that it can result in loss of the abdominal reflexes, so if they are unilaterally absent it can provide valuable information. The levels of the upper are T9 and T10 and lower, T11 and T12.
  - Hoffman's sign – in UMN lesions there is a generalised sensitivity to stretch in many muscles. Flicking the terminal phalanx of the index finger causes reflex flexion of the remaining digits.
  - The primitive reflexes indicate frontal lobe damage:
    - glabellar – tap between the eyes (from behind so they cannot see your hand); it is positive if blinking is persistent; however, it is unreliable and often unpleasant for patients
    - snout reflex – tapping the nose induces grimacing
    - sucking reflex – stroking the lips produces pouting and sucking movements of the lips
    - chewing reflex – a tongue depressor placed in the mouth produces reflex chewing
    - grasp reflex – stroking the palm elicits a grasp which gets firmer as attempts are made to remove your fingers.

Coordination

- Poor coordination can be difficult to demonstrate if the patient is weak.
  - Finger–nose testing – hold the object at the extreme of their reach and ask them to touch it and then their nose repeatedly, as accurately (not quickly) as possible. In essential tremor, the tremor on maintaining movement may persist on movement and even worsen towards an object, but only with cerebellar disease does it appear only as the hand approaches the target and true past-pointing occur.
  - Dysdiadochokinesis – failure to perform alternate movements. Thus ask them to tap one palm alternately with the palm and the dorsum of the other hand, listen to the rhythm. It is natural for the non-dominant hand to be a little less coordinated.

Sensation

- Test the following dermatomes in the upper limb (for the same modalities as in the lower limb): C5 (shoulder), C6 (lateral forearm, thumb and index finger), C7 (middle finger), C8 (little finger and lateral hand), T1 (medial forearm), T2 (medial arm).
- Test as in the lower limbs for dorsal column and spinothalamic tracts.
- The common peripheral nerve lesions likely to be encountered in PACES are discussed in Scenario 4, *Peripheral neuropathy*.
- Sensory levels on the trunk are – umbilicus T10, nipple T5. Do not forget that posteriorly in the midline L1 is obviously just below the ribcage.

EXAMINATION OF SPEECH

- For patients with a speech disturbance, speaking is a great effort and they can become easily distressed. Sit with them, and make a great effort to put them at their ease. If they start to struggle make it clear you appreciate how difficult it is for them.
- They may be reluctant to talk; engage them on a topic they can talk freely on, e.g. their holidays or job. If they are still reluctant, show them a picture in the paper and ask them to describe it. You will know what it shows.
- You are likely to meet one of two patterns: dysarthria and aphasia.
- Dysarthria – the language content is normal but articulation is troublesome:

- Repetition – difficult words, e.g. constitution, constabulary, artillery, statistical analysis. Use words of increasing complexity, e.g. city, citizen, citizenship. Test the different muscles of articulation, i.e. 'puh' – lips, 'tuh' – tongue, 'kah' – pharynx.
- Cough – a bovine cough is heard in recurrent laryngeal nerve palsy.
- Examine the motor system – is the dysarthria due to:
  - LMN weakness – facial palsy, bulbar palsy
  - UMN weakness – hemiparesis, pseudobulbar palsy
  - cerebellar disease – nystagmus, intention tremor, hypotonia and ataxia
  - extrapyramidal disease – Parkinson's disease
  - are they also dysphasic?
- Aphasia – a problem with the production or understanding of language, written, spoken or read. It signifies a problem in the dominant hemisphere. Is there a non-fluent or fluent aphasia?
  - Non-fluent – frontal lobe damage (Broca's area) causing an expressive or motor aphasia. The content may be good, but the patient says little; or if they say a lot the speech lacks a normal rhythm, with short sentences and no filler words like 'to', 'but', 'so', 'the'. For example, 'phone daughter evening'.
  - Fluent – parietal lobe damage (Wernicke's area) causing a receptive or sensory aphasia. They may talk freely, with a normal rhythm, but the content is poor. They may perform paraphasic errors, i.e. substitute consonants or words or invented words (neologisms).
  - Repetition – ask the patient to repeat the following phrase 'no ifs, ands or buts'. This confirms they are aphasic. Is comprehension normal? Body language and behaviour may be normal as they watch those around them. They may not have the words to demonstrate comprehension; thus make the answers to your questions simple: 'Are you in hospital?', 'Is my shirt blue?' They have a 50:50 chance of success and perseveration is common. Have them obey commands: 'Touch your nose', 'Lift your right hand'. Often multistep commands prove troublesome: 'Touch your head, then knee, then ear.'
    - when testing comprehension do not look at the part of the body as this may be all the clue the patient needs.
  - Describe the aphasia in terms of fluency, paraphasia, repetition and comprehension.
  - Ask them to read and write: the same patterns will be seen in their writing.
  - Check for associated neurology, e.g. weakness of the right arm or a right hemiparesis in a non-fluent aphasia, or a right homonymous hemianopia in a fluent aphasia.

STATION

Neurological Scenarios

1. Spastic paraparesis
2. Hemiparesis
3. Motor neurone disease
4. Peripheral neuropathy:
   4A Distal bilateral sensorimotor neuropathy
   4B Carpal tunnel syndrome
   4C Ulnar nerve compression at the elbow
   4D Radial nerve palsy
   4E Common peroneal nerve palsy
   4F Guillain–Barré syndrome
5. Cerebellar syndrome
6. Parkinson's disease
7. Cervical myelopathy
8. Dystrophia myotonica
9. Hereditary motor sensory neuropathy types I and II
10. Myasthenia gravis
11. Facial palsy
12. Ptosis
13. Nystagmus

1. SPASTIC PARAPARESIS

Points in the examination

- Characteristic gait
- Increased tone in the lower limbs with relatively preserved muscle bulk
- Clonus
- Weakness – symmetrical, proximal and distal; flexion > extension
- Contractures (possibly)
- Hyperreflexia with extensor plantars
- Check for sensory loss and a level, cerebellar signs and for local spinal tenderness

Aetiology

- The hypertonia, clonus and hyperreflexia tell you that the lesion lies above L1 as the pyramidal tracts end there.
- Cord compression – must always be considered. Any sensory level must always be determined, particularly if the history suggests an acute or subacute onset with recent alteration in sphincter function.
- Motor neurone disease – a complete absence of sensory signs with a combination of upper and lower motor neurone features is almost diagnostic.
- Multiple sclerosis – cerebellar signs, sensory loss (more commonly the dorsal columns than spinothalamic tract), brisk reflexes in the upper limbs, paraesthesias on flexing the neck (Lhermitte's sign), papillitis or optic atrophy, disinhibition and mention of sphincter disturbance or impotence may point to this diagnosis.
- Trauma – look for evidence of a previous injury to the spine or deformities.
- Cerebral palsy – check for intellectual impairment and behavioural problems, or a history of birth injury.

Cord lesions

These are either intrinsic or extrinsic:
- Extrinsic – lesions which are important from a therapeutic point of view are usually one of the 'three Ts' – tumours (primary or secondary), tubercle (occasionally other infections) or trauma (including spondylosis).
- Intrinsic – vitamin B_{12} deficiency, being treatable, is the most important intrinsic lesion and demyelination the most common.

Aetiology related to onset of paraparesis

Acute or subacute

- Disc prolapse above L1–L2
- Tumours:
  - Intra- and extradural; carcinoma (lung, breast, kidney and prostate), lymphoma, myeloma or leukaemia; the commonest benign lesions are thoracic meningiomas and neurofibromas
- Cervical spondylosis
- Infection:
  - Abscess, syphilitic myelitis, HIV infection, Pott's disease of the spine
- Rheumatoid arthritis – atlantoaxial subluxation
- Haemorrhage:
  - Any cause of thrombocytopenia, or bleeding diathesis, arteriovenous malformation (AVM), primary intramedullary haemorrhage
- Vascular:
  - Arterial occlusion – thrombotic, embolic, dissection, vasculitic, hypotensive
- Inflammatory:
  - Sarcoid, SLE, multiple sclerosis, transverse myelitis
- Subacute combined degeneration of the cord

Chronic

- Multiple sclerosis
- Motor neurone disease
- Syringomyelia
- Primary intramedullary and dural tumours, or indeed any cause of compression
- Human T-cell leukaemia virus-1 (HTLV-1) – tropical spastic paraparesis
- Radiation myelopathy
- Subacute combined degeneration of the cord

Symptoms

- Weakness of the lower limbs is the most common.
- Key questions to determine the aetiology are duration of onset, sphincter disturbance and associated features of the underlying cause.

Investigations

- Suspicion of spinal cord compression is a medical emergency. Once sphincter dysfunction has been present for 24 hours, it is irreversible. Therefore the necessary investigations must be carried out as a matter of urgency – FBC, ESR, CXR, plain radiology of the spine, then either a CT myelogram or MRI. A neurosurgeon should be contacted.
- Depending on the likely differential diagnosis:
  - Electromyography
  - Nerve conduction studies
  - Lumbar puncture – CSF for oligoclonal bands, culture, acid-fast bacilli, ACE and cytospin
  - Blood and CSF syphilis serology
  - Blood culture
  - Biopsy of masses
  - HIV test
  - Vitamin B_{12} levels, CRP, autoantibodies and MRI of the central nervous system.

Management

- This is dependent on the cause.
- Spinal cord compression with bladder or bowel involvement often requires surgical decompression. Stabilisation of the spine may be necessary. Dexamethasone and radiotherapy may suffice for malignant compression.
- The main problem with benign tumours is that the paraparesis may be attributed to multiple sclerosis, despite the symptoms not being disseminated in time and place. With malignancy the main danger is indecision: the condition is obviously incurable but surgical treatment at an early stage may relieve pain, minimise weakness and preserve bladder function.

Points of interest

- Lesions below L1 can result in cauda equina compression (see p. 216).
- This too is a medical emergency:
    - Flaccid paraparesis
    - Saddle anaesthesia
    - Reduced reflexes
    - Downgoing plantars
    - Sphincter disturbance.

2. HEMIPARESIS

Points in the examination

Only on the affected side of the body:
- Characteristic gait.
- Paucity of movement.
- Pyramidal posture – the upper limb tends to be flexed at the elbow, pronated and internally rotated at the shoulder, and the lower limb extended at the hip and knee, with the foot inverted and plantar-flexed.
- Pyramidal drift – perhaps the only early sign.
- Clasp-knife spasticity in a pyramidal distribution ± clonus.
- Weakness or paralysis in a pyramidal distribution.
- Hyperreflexia, upgoing plantars (Babinski's sign), and Hoffman's reflex.
- Weakness in the motor divisions of the cranial nerves ± a homonymous quadrantanopia/hemianopia; there may be papilloedema.
- Check for a gag reflex on both sides of the palate.
- If the postcentral gyrus is involved, or the internal capsule, there may be hemisensory loss, or just sensory inattention.
- Dysphasia:
  - Broca's area – anterior lesions causing an expressive dysphasia with non-fluent speech but intact understanding; the patient should be asked to write or even sing
  - Wernicke's area – posterior lesions causing a receptive dysphasia can be difficult to identify; the speech is fluent but mistakes made in syllables, to talking fluent nonsense can occur; there is little or no understanding and 'confusion' is often an erroneous diagnosis.

Aetiology (in the contralateral hemisphere)

- Stroke:
  - Ischaemic:
    - cardiovascular disease and risk factors, prothrombotic tendencies, vasculitis, internal carotid artery dissection, foci for emboli – cardiac (e.g. AF, mural thrombus, subacute bacterial endocarditis (SBE)) or peripheral, through a patent foramen ovale

- Haemorrhagic:
  - hypertension, aneurysm (e.g. SAH), AVM, thrombocytopenia or bleeding diatheses
- Space-occupying lesion in the cranium:
  - tumour, aneurysm, abscess, haematoma, granuloma, tuberculoma, toxoplasmoma, cysts (e.g. cysticercosis)

Symptoms

The duration of onset is crucial for the differential diagnosis.
- An abrupt onset of neurological deficit with a tendency to improve, with or without preceding transient ischaemia, in the presence of cardiovascular risk factors, is almost diagnostic of stroke.
- A protracted history with a slowly worsening circadian headache, drowsiness, vomiting, symptoms attributable to focal brain damage and seizures suggests a space-occupying lesion. The nature of the lesion usually dictates the speed of onset, e.g. meningioma or breast carcinoma metastases.

Initial investigations

- FBC, ESR, glucose and lipids, clotting, U+E.
- CXR.
- ECG.
- As 80–90% of strokes are ischaemic a CT brain is not always necessary for the diagnosis:
  - However, it is definitely indicated if there is any suggestion of an intracranial haemorrhage or doubt about the aetiology, e.g. subdural haematoma, tumour and intracranial infection can all mimic stroke
  - In practice, most stroke patients have a CT brain scan.
- If there is suspicion of cerebellar or brainstem disease a CT is necessary, as swelling in the posterior fossa can be rapidly life-threatening. CT ± contrast will identify a mass lesion.

Further investigations

- Thrombophilia screen – protein C and S, antithrombin III, activated protein C ratio, lupus anticoagulant, VDRL (Venereal Disease Research Laboratory – test for syphilis), factor V Leiden mutation and prothrombin mutation.
- ANA, dsDNA, C3, C4 – vasculitis.

- Echo.
- Carotid Doppler ultrasound.
- MRI may help to classify mass lesions and reveal evidence of more diffuse disease; it is preferable to CT for examination of the posterior fossa.
- MR angiography – delineates extracranial arterial disease (internal carotid artery dissection must be considered in young patients) and proximal intracranial arteries, and detects thrombosis of major cerebral veins, venous sinuses and aneurysms.
- Lumbar puncture if low-grade meningitis suspected, after CT, as the presence of focal signs necessitates exclusion of raised intracranial pressure.
- Search for a primary focus of malignancy or infection, or a cause of immunosuppression in space-occupying lesions.

Management

Stroke

- Adequate oxygenation, hydration, cautious attention to hypertension if severe and control of blood glucose are important initially.
- Prevention of secondary morbidity and mortality from cardiovascular disease is paramount; attention must be paid to all risk factors.
- Stroke units with dedicated multidisciplinary teams are beneficial for preventing early and late mortality and improving functional ability.
- Identify patients who will benefit from anticoagulation (cf. AF) or endarterectomy in the early period.
- Patients who receive thrombolysis within 6 hours of the onset of an ischaemic stroke have a better prognosis. CT may identify those less likely to benefit. This is currently not routine practice in the UK.
- Intracranial haemorrhage requires an urgent neurosurgical opinion.
- Space-occupying lesions should be excised if possible. Analgesia for headache, dexamethasone ± mannitol for oedema.

3. MOTOR NEURONE DISEASE

Points in the examination

Any combination of upper and lower motor neurone symptoms and signs, often asymmetrical initially. Three clinical patterns are initially seen which tend to merge with time:

- Amyotrophic lateral sclerosis (ALS):
  - Spastic tetraparesis or paraparesis (lateral corticospinal tracts) with added lower motor neurone signs – wasting and fasciculation (anterior horn cells). NB. ALS often initially presents with predominant spinal UMN signs – primary lateral sclerosis.
- Progressive muscular atrophy:
  - Predominant lower motor neurone signs in the limbs, particularly wasting, fasciculation and weakness in the hands and arms.
- Bulbar palsy:
  - LMN involvement of the lower cranial nerves – dysarthria with quiet, hoarse or nasal speech, palsy of the muscles of mastication, facial muscles, muscles of deglutition and the tongue, which is flaccid and shows fasciculation
  - The jaw jerk is normal or absent and the gag reflex is diminished or absent (in contrast to pseudobulbar palsy – an UMN lesion, with a small spastic tongue and exaggerated jaw jerk and gag reflex. It can coexist in MND but is rarer).

Aetiology

- There are familial and sporadic forms of ALS. In 20% of familial forms there is an identifiable mutation in the gene for copper/zinc superoxide dismutase-1 (SOD-1) located on the long arm of chromosome 21. Genotype and phenotype correlate poorly. In the majority of cases, however, the cause is unknown.
- It is rare and tends to affect middle-aged to elderly people.

Symptoms

- Bulbar – dysarthria and dysphonia, dysphagia and difficulty chewing with nasal regurgitation of fluids, recurrent chest infections and dyspnoea (orthopnoea due to diaphragmatic weakness).
- Limbs – weakness of a hand or the whole upper limb, with wasting that the patient has noticed (the muscles may appear to have been sucked out of the hand), progressive foot drop; cramps are common.

Differential diagnosis

- MS – no sensory abnormality in MND
- Polyneuropathies – no sensory abnormality in MND
- Cervical myelopathy – if no cranial nerve signs
- Motor neuropathy – if limb signs are entirely LMN
- Cord or cauda-equina compression – cause sphincter disturbance which does not occur in MND
- Myasthenia gravis – weakness of the external ocular muscles does not occur in MND
- Diabetic amyotrophy – proximal lower limb weakness and wasting
- Cervical and lumbar stenosis – this combination may cause UMN signs in the upper limbs and LMN signs in the lower limbs

Investigations

- The diagnosis is clinical, and depends on the simultaneous existence of UMN and LMN signs in the same muscle groups in the limbs and similar signs affecting the cranial nerve innervated muscles.
- If there is any concern that a spinal cord lesion might be present, imaging of the spine is essential, ideally MRI.
- Electromyography (EMG) will show denervation but not the cause, surface EMG in all limbs can reveal widespread denervation before signs.

Management

- Mostly supportive, the aim is to overcome difficulties and reduce symptoms. Speech therapy may help with dysarthria, dysphonia and dysphagia.
- It has a remorseless progression, with death usually occurring within 2–4 years of diagnosis.

- Riluzole has been recommended by NICE for asymptomatic patients with amyotrophic lateral sclerosis; it extends the time to mechanical ventilation in this invariably fatal disease.

4. PERIPHERAL NEUROPATHY

A number of different cases of peripheral neuropathy may be encountered in the examination.

To aid in determining the aetiology the following questions should be considered:
- Is it a symmetrical polyneuropathy, mononeuropathy or mononeuritis multiplex?
  - In general, toxic and metabolic nerve disorders produce a symmetrical syndrome. Asymmetrical involvement of one or more nerves suggests local compression, entrapment or local infarction of the nerve or nerves secondary to disease of the nutrient vessels.
- Is it primarily motor, sensory or mixed?
  - Most symptoms and signs suggest mixed, but motor predominates in Guillain–Barré syndrome, porphyria and lead poisoning (rare). By contrast, hereditary sensory neuropathy, vitamin B_{12} deficiency and some carcinomas of the lung predominantly affect the sensory system.
- Is there a history of occupational or recreational exposure to toxins, most commonly alcohol?
- Are there associated symptoms of systemic disease, e.g. diabetes mellitus, hypothyroidism, renal failure, malignant disease, collagen vascular disease, pernicious anaemia?
- Is there a family history?
  - Most commonly, hereditary motor sensory neuropathy (HMSN) types-1 and -2, which used to be called 'Charcot–Marie–Tooth disease' or 'peroneal muscular atrophy'.

The following cases may be seen.

4A PERIPHERAL NEUROPATHY – DISTAL BILATERAL SENSORIMOTOR NEUROPATHY

Points in the examination

- Stocking/glove sensory loss
- Loss of tendon reflexes
- Weakness of the hip girdle and shoulder girdle
- Look for ulcers or Charcot's joints

Aetiology

- Metabolic, e.g. diabetes mellitus, uraemia, hypothyroidism, porphyria, amyloidosis
- Malignant disease
- Collagen vascular disease, e.g. SLE, rheumatoid arthritis (RA), polyarteritis nodosa (PAN), scleroderma
- Deficiencies, e.g. vitamin B_{12} and folate, thiamine (Wernicke's encephalopathy and Korsakoff's psychosis in alcoholics) and niacin (pellagra)
- Inflammatory, e.g. Guillain–Barré syndrome, leprosy or diphtheria
- Toxic, e.g. alcohol, drugs (isoniazid, vincristine, amiodarone, cisplatin), heavy metals
- Hereditary, e.g. HMSN-1 and -2, Refsum's disease, Friedreich's ataxia

Symptoms

The following apply typically to patients with diabetes:
- Unpleasant tingling, numbness, burning and aching in the lower legs and feet, mild weakness, nocturnal discomfort, progression over many months.
- Painless, punched out, plantar foot ulcers are seen and are a major cause of morbidity.
- The following are associated with diabetic neuropathy and may be sought if warranted:
  - Autonomic dysfunction – impotence, urinary retention, diarrhoea, constipation, postural hypotension (prudent and simple to check for)
  - Amyotrophy – proximal weakness, weight loss, slight sensory signs

- Femoral/sciatic neuralgia – NB. In diabetic sciatic neuropathy straight leg raise is normal and Lasègue's sign is absent
- Thoracic radiculopathy.

Investigations

- They are directed (by the pattern of the presentation) at the underlying cause for the precise diagnosis, but nerve conduction studies ± EMG can be helpful. Where there is a segmental demyelination, e.g. in diabetes, carcinoma or Guillain–Barré syndrome (GBS), abnormalities are detected with ease, but in an axonal degeneration, e.g. alcohol, the overall conduction velocity can remain normal despite a reduction in the number of units.
- Fasting glucose, serum vitamin B_{12}, protein electrophoresis, ESR, FBC, U+E, bone profile, LFT and γ-GT, CXR, LP (in GBS shows raised protein level).
- Nerve biopsy in progressive neuropathy or to identify vasculitis as a cause. Sensory nerves are usually biopsied.

Management

- Directed towards the specific cause.
- Rigorous control of glycaemia, often with intensive insulin regimes, can improve diabetic neuropathy, particularly if the syndrome arose acutely. Simple analgesics, tricyclic antidepressants, anticonvulsants (phenytoin and carbamazepine), oral mexiletine, intravenous lidocaine (lignocaine) or topical capsaicin may be helpful.
- Autonomic neuropathy is difficult:
  - Postural hypotension – helped by raising the head of the bed at night or fludrocortisone
  - Vomiting – metoclopramide
  - Erythromycin or tetracycline are used to cure the bacterial overgrowth responsible for diarrhoea
  - Impotence may require vacuum devices, intracavernosal papaverine or prostaglandin E_1 (also intraurethral) or sildenafil (Viagra).
- In nutritional deficiency, replace:
  - Subacute combined degeneration of the cord (SCDC), if suspected, demands emergency treatment with intramuscular vitamin B_{12}
  - Incipient iron deficiency can be revealed with B_{12} therapy.
- SCDC can be precipitated by giving folate to treat megaloblastic anaemia where vitamin B_{12} deficiency is present. Thus B_{12} deficiency must be excluded.

4B PERIPHERAL NEUROPATHY – CARPAL TUNNEL SYNDROME

Points in the examination

- Decreased sensation in the median nerve distribution:
  - Light touch and two-point discrimination are most affected. Pinprick and heat/cold are less often impaired. Joint proprioception is preserved.
- The palm is spared as the palmar branch of the nerve lies superior to the retinaculum.
- If prolonged:
  - Wasting of the outer thenar eminence
  - Weakness of abductor pollicis brevis and opponens pollicis can be demonstrated.
- Tinel's and Phalen's signs may be positive (but have no predictive value for the presence or absence of median nerve compression).
- Are there scars over the carpal tunnels?
- Look for features of an underlying cause (see Aetiology, below).
- Beware of a cervical radiculopathy.

Aetiology

- Usually idiopathic or related to repeated occupational trauma.
- Pregnancy, rheumatoid arthritis, hypothyroidism, acromegaly, gout, menopause.

Symptoms

- Pain and tingling and eventually decreased sensation in the thumb, index, middle and radial half of the ring fingers. Symptoms may be more proximal, even up to the arm in some. It is worse at night, or first thing in the morning, and may be relieved by shaking the hand at one's side.

Management

- Rest, splinting, diuretics and local hydrocortisone injection may help temporarily while an underlying cause is relieved.
- Division of the flexor retinaculum will rapidly relieve symptoms. Sensory function will return over 6–12 months and muscle power, if impaired, may return almost to normal.

4C PERIPHERAL NEUROPATHY – ULNAR NERVE COMPRESSION AT THE ELBOW

Points in the examination

- Wasting of flexor carpi ulnaris and flexor digitorum profundus may be seen on the inner aspect of the flexor surface of the forearm.
- Hand deviates to the radial side on flexion of the wrist against resistance.
- Hypothenar eminence, interossei and ulnar half of thenar eminence wasting.
- Hyperextension of the metacarpophalangeal joints in the little and ring fingers with flexion of their interphalangeal joints – the ulnar claw hand.
- The adductors and abductors are paralysed – one must examine the hand with the palm pressed against a flat surface as, to some extent, the long extensors and flexors act as abductors and adductors.
- Adductor pollicis is weak – ask the patient to hold a piece of paper between the thumb and index finger; the thumb will flex in an ulnar nerve palsy (Froment's sign).
- Sensory loss over the little and medial half of the ring finger.
- Evidence of surgery, osteoarthritis (OA) or fracture at the elbow.

Aetiology/symptoms and management

- Damage to the nerve in the ulnar groove at the elbow – pressure, fracture or OA.
- Sensory symptoms are not prominent, but the patient may notice some numbness and tingling of the two ulnar fingers and the ulnar border of the palm. Usually attention is drawn to the palm by the muscular wasting and weakness.
- Change habits if they are responsible, or release the nerve from the ulnar groove and place anteriorly.

4D PERIPHERAL NEUROPATHY – RADIAL NERVE PALSY

Points in the examination

- Look for wrist drop and weakness of finger extension.
- If triceps is spared but the extensors in the forearm and the extensors of the thumb are wasted and weak, it is likely the nerve is damaged in the spiral groove of the humerus – 'Saturday night palsy'.
- If triceps is also involved it is likely the damage occurred in or above the axilla.
- NB. Wrist drop due to lead poisoning is a historical rarity.
- Sensory loss is variable and may be absent.

Management

- The prognosis is good; in compression, recovery is over weeks. Even if the wrist requires splinting, muscle function starts to recover 4–8 months later.
- The wrist must be splinted in extension as must the MCP joints – the latter not rigidly.

4E PERIPHERAL NEUROPATHY – COMMON PERONEAL NERVE PALSY

Points in the examination

$(L_5 L_1)$

(ankle jerk)

- Foot drop.
- Wasting of peronei and anterior tibial muscles.
- Loss of eversion of the foot.
- Inversion is lost when the foot is dorsiflexed, but weak inversion is possible with plantarflexion.
- Sensation is impaired over the dorsum of the foot, including the first phalanges of the toes and the anterolateral aspect of the bottom half of the leg.
- The nerve is damaged as it winds round the neck of the fibula, e.g. a fracture of the head of the fibula in an inversion injury at the ankle.

Aetiology

- Damage to the nerve as it winds round the neck of the fibula, e.g. fracture
- Mononeuritis

Management

- Orthoses

4F   PERIPHERAL NEUROPATHY – GUILLAIN–BARRÉ SYNDROME

Unlikely to see this in PACES.

Points in the examination/aetiology/symptoms/ management

- Acute weakness starting in the legs, spreading rapidly (few days) to involve muscles of the arms and trunk, occasionally preceded by tingling in the hands and feet, with bulbar and facial weakness (50%); dysphagia and dyspnoea (intercostal muscle weakness) is characteristic of the syndrome. No bladder or bowel symptoms, nor a sensory level.
- In GBS, intravenous immunoglobulin or plasma exchange is beneficial if used at the outset; 80–95% of people recover completely over several months.
- NB. In GBS (and myasthenia and – the now extremely rare – poliomyelitis), respiratory failure, which is completely treatable, can develop with alarming rapidity and patients who are ill or deteriorating must have access to a ventilator.

5. CEREBELLAR SYNDROME

Points in the examination

- Scanning, staccato (interrupted), slurred speech
- Nystagmus – usually towards the side with the lesion
- On the affected side (may be global):
  - Hypotonia
  - Hyporeflexia
  - Ataxia
  - Intention tremor and past-pointing
  - Dysdiadochokinesis
  - Gait – broad-based and unsteady; falls to affected side on walking (can be brought out on heel-to-toe walking), Romberg's test negative
- Vermal lesion may give truncal rather than limb ataxia; patients can appear perfectly well until asked to stand

Aetiology

A lesion in the ipsilateral cerebellar hemisphere:
- Multiple sclerosis
- Cerebellar or brainstem stroke – thromboembolic or haemorrhagic
- Space-occupying lesion – e. g. primary or secondary tumour
- Severe hypothyroidism
- Chronic alcohol abuse
- Phenytoin
- Paraneoplastic
- Friedreich's ataxia (autosomal recessive (AR) or X-linked, onset in childhood, always before 25 years of age: pes cavus, kyphoscoliosis, spastic paraparesis with extensor plantars, but areflexia due to an axonal neuropathy, spinocerebellar degeneration causes ataxia, diabetes mellitus in 10% of patients, some have intellectual impairment, cardiomyopathy in two-thirds of cases)
- Lesions at the cerebellopontine angle, usually an acoustic neuroma, cause ipsilateral deafness, loss of the corneal reflex, later sensory loss on the face, Vth nerve and VIIth nerve weakness; eventually brainstem compression occurs with long tract signs and hydrocephalus

Differential diagnosis

- Wilson's disease – tremor, chorea, dysarthria, mental deterioration, cirrhosis; AR (chromosome 13); see p. 51.
- Refsum's disease – pes cavus, retinitis pigmentosa, nerve deafness, anosmia, cerebellar ataxia; AR – due to abnormality in lipid metabolism – excess phytanic acid.
- Both are treatable diseases which may present with ataxia.

Symptoms

- Headache – many patients, even some with large tumours, present with a mild but persistent occipital headache, worse in the morning and recurs on straining. As intracranial pressure rises, the headache becomes severe and generalised with associated impairment of vision (papilloedema may occur).
- Visceral disturbances – persistent vomiting, hiccup, cardiorespiratory dysfunction and sudden death occur in patients with this group of tumours.
- Cranial nerve dysfunction arises from compression of the brainstem nuclei.
- Hydrocephalus – dilatation of the lateral ventricles, especially the frontal horns, can cause intellectual and behavioural impairment.

Investigations

- MRI posterior fossa (or CT if MRI unavailable); even with trivial symptoms and signs there can be a considerable mass in the posterior fossa; many are cystic and amenable to surgery
- LP if there is no space-occupying lesion
- Phenytoin level
- Blood alcohol, LFT, γ-GT
- TSH, T_4
- Glucose, lipids
- HIV test
- CXR – lung cancer causing paraneoplastic syndrome, or with multiple metastases
- ECG

Management

- Excision or evacuation of posterior fossa masses if possible, shunting for hydrocephalus. Radiotherapy has a role in selected cases.
- Ensure abstinence from alcohol.
- Give thyroxine replacement.
- Reduce phenytoin dose.

6. PARKINSON'S DISEASE

Points in the examination

Classic trilogy is resting tremor, bradykinesia and rigidity.
- Resting, 'pill-rolling' tremor or on maintained posture
- Bradykinesia – difficulty initiating movements and poverty of movement:
  - Mask-like facies
  - Dysarthria, quiet monotonous voice
  - Festinant, small-paced gait, no arm swinging, difficulty turning
  - Dribbling of saliva
  - Impaired writing (micrographia) and dressing ability
- Stooped, flexed posture, difficulty maintaining posture
- Tendency to fall if standing still
- Lead-pipe rigidity with cogwheeling (tremor superimposed on rigidity)
- Look for other neurological features of the 'Parkinson's plus' syndromes:
  - Multisystem atrophy – autonomic failure (Shy–Drager), ataxia (olivopontocerebellar degeneration) and severe akinesia (striatonigral degeneration)
  - Progressive supranuclear palsy – failure of downward gaze, pyramidal signs and dementia (Steele–Richardson–Olszweski syndrome)

Symptoms

- Tremor, usually asymmetrical, very common
- Bradykinesia is usually not noticed by the patient but commented on by the relatives; often the most disabling feature
- Postural abnormalities and difficulty in walking can lead to instability and falls
- Constipation
- Depression

Aetiology

- Unknown, but probably reflects a genetic susceptibility to environmental factors.
- Causes destruction of the dopaminergic neurones in the substantia nigra. About 85% of these neurones must be lost, with a corresponding loss of dopamine, before symptoms and signs occur.
- The median age of onset is 55 years.

Differential diagnosis

- Parkinsonism (as opposed to Parkinson's disease) is seen in the following situations:
  - Pure parkinsonism:
    - postencephalitic parkinsonism (encephalitis lethargica)
    - neuroleptic drugs
    - MPTP (1-methyl-4-phenyl-1,2,3,6-tetrahydropyridine) toxicity
    - cerebral anoxia, due to bilateral basal ganglia infarction
  - Parkinsonism with other neurological features:
    - Wilson's disease
    - Huntington's chorea
    - cerebral palsy
    - progressive supranuclear palsy (Steele–Richardson–Olszewski syndrome)
    - multisystem atrophy (Shy–Drager)
    - cortical Lewy body disease.
- See *Tremor*, p. 212.

Investigations

- There is no diagnostic test. Diagnosis is clinical and needs the presence of two out of the features of bradykinesia, rigidity and tremor. The response to pharmacological therapy confirms Parkinson's disease. If there is no response to therapy consider the differential diagnoses.

Management

- Levodopa – the 'gold standard' of treatment, but it may be associated with an earlier onset of motor fluctuations; thus it may be preferable to delay its use, particularly in younger patients. In older patients and in those with significant disability it should not be delayed. It is combined with the dopa-decarboxylase inhibitors, benserazide and carbidopa.

- Dopamine agonist monotherapy with ropinirole may delay the onset of motor fluctuations. Other class members include the ergot derivatives, apomorphine and pramipexole.
- The role of selegiline in neuroprotection remains controversial. Entacapone and amantadine have a role.
- Antimuscarinics reduce cholinergic activity in the brain, and are particularly useful for drug-induced or post-encephalitic parkinsonism.
- Surgical therapies such as pallidotomy, bilateral subthalamic deep-brain stimulation and fetal-tissue transplantation can be considered for those who fail medical therapy.

7. CERVICAL MYELOPATHY

Points in the examination

- In the lower limbs – clasp-knife spasticity, with preserved bulk
- Clonus at the ankle ± knee
- Weakness – in a pyramidal distribution
- Hyperreflexia – in the lower limbs, Babinski's sign
- Dorsal column (vibration and cutaneous sensation before proprioception) or spinothalamic loss
- Loss of abdominal reflexes
- In the upper limbs – often asymmetrical reflexes, inverted reflexes (see opposite) or the mid-cervical reflex pattern (see opposite)
- The signs in the upper limbs are often not marked; wasting of the small muscles does not occur unless there is a radiculopathy affecting C8 or T1

Symptoms

- Chronic weakness of the lower limbs and loss of sensation; the latter may continue up the trunk.
- Bladder or bowel disturbance occurs (although not always), and in men loss of potency.
- Sensory symptoms in the lower limbs, up the trunk or in the upper limbs are not always present, even with clear signs.
- Painful cervical spine, but not always, with reduced movements.

Aetiology

- Cervical spondylosis – degenerative disease is most pronounced in the mid-cervical region at C5/6, and the myelopathy associated with spondylosis is often maximal at this level.

Differential diagnosis

- The commonest causes of a cervical cord lesion are cervical spondylosis and demyelination, although tumours – both intrinsic and extrinsic – and syringomyelia need consideration. The duration of onset and associated features are helpful.
- Demyelination – other lesions dissociated in space.
- Syringomyelia – dissociated sensory loss ± bulbar signs.

Intrinsic cord lesions – spinothalamic loss occurs earlier than dorsal column loss.

Investigations

- Clinical differentiation between the causes and particularly exclusion of a tumour is not usually possible, thus the cord needs imaging. The signs in the upper limb and the sensory level help dictate where the spine is imaged. MRI is the ideal investigation or CT myelography.
- Measure vitamin B_{12}.

Management

- Myelopathy at one level if due to a disc prolapse, or multiple levels due to diffuse narrowing of the canal, are best managed in consultation with a neurosurgeon.
- Conservative management with a collar, only if surgery is unsuitable.

Points of interest

- Inverted reflexes are the extension of triceps when the biceps is tapped and finger flexion when supinator is tapped. Biceps and supinator jerks may be absent due to damage at C5/6, whereas the triceps and finger jerks are brisk because their reflex arcs lie below the level of the lesion. This is the mid-cervical reflex pattern.

8. DYSTROPHIA MYOTONICA

Points in the examination

- Long, expressionless face
- Ptosis – bilateral
- Wasting of temporalis, masseter and invariably sternomastoid
- Frontal baldness in men
- Cataracts
- Myotonia:
  - Difficulty in releasing grip, e.g. on handshake
  - Percussion myotonia – best seen in the tongue (as teeth marks) or at the thenar eminence
- Dystrophy:
  - Wasting and weakness of the peripheral muscles, initially distal (forearms especially, sparing the small muscles of the hands) but subsequently proximal and limb-girdle
  - Hyporeflexia and subsequent areflexia develop
  - Myotonia may disappear as weakness develops
  - External ophthalmoplegia (rare)
  - Dysphagia and dysarthria develop from both weakness and incoordination consequent on myotonia
- Reduced intelligence or progressive dementia
- Bradycardia and cardiomegaly may occur
- Pacemaker
- Cor pulmonale secondary to diaphragmatic weakness, with subsequent hypoxaemia, or right heart failure
- The testicles are small and firm
- Gynaecomastia

Aetiology

- Inherited as an autosomal dominant condition, the locus is at chromosome 19 q13.2–q13.3. Males > females.
- Exhibits anticipation, whereby the features become more severe and appear earlier in subsequent generations. Presenile cataracts may have been present in prior generations before the full-blown syndrome occurs in an individual. There may have been a progressive social decline in the family in successive generations.
- Diabetes mellitus occurs in 5% of cases due to impaired insulin secretion.

- The cardiac disorder occurs in two-thirds of cases, most often recognised on ECG rather than clinically. It is due to disease of the conducting system rather than of the myocardium.

Differential diagnosis

- Facioscapulohumeral dystrophy – facial, neck and upper limb-girdle wasting; deltoid hypertrophy; winging of the scapulas; absent UL reflexes; no myotonia, balding or gonadal failure; younger onset; intelligence is normal
- Limb-girdle dystrophy – this autosomal recessive disease does not cause facial weakness and wasting, but predominantly shoulder weakness
- Hypothyroidism – slowness of thought, and prolonged muscular contraction (see p. 408)

Symptoms

- Presentation is in the third and fourth decades, often after the gene has been passed on, before the onset of gonadal failure.
- Weakness of the hands and difficulty walking are the usual initial symptoms.
- Myotonia is rarely obtrusive initially, but the failure to release grip can become troublesome. Myotonia is often worse when cold or excited.
- Poor vision, weight loss, impotence, ptosis and increased sweating are common.
- Later in the course of the disease, low-output heart failure consequent on bradycardia/heart block, and hypersomnolence occurs.
- Stokes–Adams attacks can occur.
- Death usually results from cardiorespiratory failure in middle age, within 15–20 years of the onset.

Investigations

- Creatinine kinase – can be raised 2–10 times normal
- IgG – reduced due to excess catabolism
- TSH, T_4
- FSH raised due to gonadal resistance; normal testosterone
- ECG – low-voltage P waves, bradycardia, first-degree block or more complex disorders

- Electromyography – demonstrate myotonic discharges evoked by movement of the electrode; myopathic potentials are recorded from weakened and wasted muscles during volitional movement:
  - EMG will exclude McArdle's disease where painful and reversible contractures occur after exertion due to myophosphorylase deficiency, and cases of polymyositis, polyneuropathy and spinal muscular atrophy where percussion myotonia can rarely occur
- Muscle biopsy – frequent long chains of nuclei are seen in the middle of muscle fibres; these changes are much more marked postmortem

Management

- No treatment influences the progressive muscle wasting and weakness that eventually develops.
- Myotonia itself can be treated, but only if it causes functional impairment, with procainamide and/or phenytoin.
- Fit a pacemaker for symptomatic bradycardia.

9. HEREDITARY MOTOR SENSORY NEUROPATHY (HMSN) TYPES I AND II (CHARCOT–MARIE–TOOTH DISEASE OR PERONEAL MUSCULAR ATROPHY)

Points in the examination

Type I

- Pes cavus with or without an equinovarus deformity and clawing of the toes.
- Kyphoscoliosis.
- Severe, symmetrical distal wasting in the legs, later in the upper limbs also; this may spare the upper part of the lower limb (in 50% cases) causing the 'inverted champagne bottle' appearance or stork legs.
- Tremor in the upper limb may occur in some cases.
- Weakness distally which tends to cause bilateral foot drop.
- Tendon reflexes are depressed or lost.
- Sensory loss distally to a variable degree may occur.
- Steppage gait.
- Ataxia may be present (this may be referred to as Roussy–Lévy syndrome, but it is not genetically distinct).
- Peripheral nerves may be thickened.

Type II

- Tends to be confined to the lower limbs.
- Wasting and weakness is less severe.
- Reflexes are absent in the lower limbs but normal in the upper limbs.
- Foot and spinal deformity are less common.
- Peripheral nerves are not palpable.

Aetiology

- Both types have an autosomal dominant pattern of inheritance; sporadic cases occur.
- Types I and II are distinct.
- Men are more severely affected than women.

Symptoms

- Type I HMSN presents in the first decade with difficulty walking or foot deformity.
- Type II HMSN has a later onset, with a peak in the second decade, but many cases present in middle or even late adult life, with weakness or wasting.

Differential diagnosis

- Peripheral neuropathy – wasting is not such a feature, sensory loss is more marked and perhaps in a stocking distribution. If the neuropathy is longstanding pes cavus may occur.
- Mononeuropathy – may occur in the context of diabetic peripheral neuropathy or vasculitis; the common peroneal nerve may be damaged at the neck of the fibula. However, mononeuropathy is neither symmetrical nor proximal.
- L4/5 root lesion – may cause bilateral foot drop but inversion at the ankle is obviously lost, with dermatomal sensory signs. Furthermore, adduction may be impaired but the reflexes are normal.
- Cauda equina lesions – must be actively considered where there are distal signs, e.g. an absent ankle jerk. There is saddle anaesthesia and sphincter involvement.
- Motor neurone disease – progressive muscular atrophy may cause LMN signs in the limbs, but the pattern of the disease, with appearance of UMN signs and the complete absence of sensory involvement, help to differentiate between the two disease processes.

Investigation

- Nerve conduction velocity is severely reduced in type I, but is either normal or only slightly reduced in type II. The reduction in conduction velocity indicates a severe demyelinating neuropathy.

Management

- Orthotic appliances and sometimes surgical correction of foot deformity or tendon transfer can help affected individuals.

10. MYASTHENIA GRAVIS

Points in the examination

- Ptosis – can be unilateral.
- The head may be held back, the patient looking down their nose to counteract the ptosis.
- Expressionless face.
- Myasthenic snarl on attempted smile.
- Muscle bulk normal early in the disease.
- Weakness and the key feature – fatiguability:
  - Ptosis develops on sustained upward gaze
  - Diplopia on holding the extremes of gaze
  - Inability to read aloud or count continually; the voice becoming quiet
  - Arm weakness proximally > distally on repeatedly lifting a weight
  - Neck weakness on holding the head up from the pillow.
- Shoulder weakness more than pelvic weakness.
- Tendon reflexes are normal.
- Sensation is normal.

Aetiology

- Unknown.
- Acquired weakness and fatiguability of muscle; the heart is uninvolved.
- It may be localised or generalised, and is due to a defect of transmission at the neuromuscular junction.
- IgG antibodies to the acetylcholine receptor are found. Immune complexes (IgG and complement) are deposited at the postsynaptic membrane that cause interference and subsequent destruction of the acetylcholine receptor.
- Thymic hyperplasia is present in 70% of patients under 40 years of age. These patients have an increased association with HLA B8 and DR3.
- Thymic tumours occur in 10%, the incidence increases with age. These patients have antibodies to striated muscle.
- Peak incidence is in the 4th decade.
- Women are affected twice as often as men.
- It may be associated with other organ- and non-organ-specific autoimmune diseases, e.g. thyroid dysfunction, rheumatoid arthritis, pernicious anaemia and SLE.

Symptoms

- The complaint of weakness on work or the prospect of work is common, but objective weakness on exertion, relieved by rest, is rare: this is the hallmark of myasthenia gravis.
- The commonest initial presentation is weakness, often affecting only the extraocular muscles, usually with ptosis – ocular myasthenia. It may only cause diplopia at the end of the day.
- The proximal limb muscles, the muscles of mastication, speech and facial expression are those commonly affected in the early stages.
- Bulbar weakness can lead to the regurgitation of fluids.
- Respiratory weakness may occur.
- It may be very localised at the outset but becomes generalised with time.
- It tends to relapse and remit, and intercurrent illness, particularly infection, may provoke severe exacerbations.
- Pregnancy, hypokalaemia, overtreatment, change of climate, extreme emotion, exercise and certain drugs, e.g. penicillamine, opiates, aminoglycosides, suxamethonium, β-blockers, can also provoke deterioration.

Investigations

- The diagnosis can be made clinically in many cases.
- Acetylcholine receptor antibodies – 90% sensitivity, 100% specificity, such that usually you do not have to resort to a Tensilon® test. (Two syringes are prepared, one with 10 ml normal saline, the other with 10 mg edrophonium diluted to 10 ml. A blinded observer must comment on the effect of a test dose of 2 ml of each IV injection (reactions can occur so resuscitation facilities, with atropine, must be present). After 30 s give the remainder of both. The observer comments on the effect of both. It is positive if only edrophonium improves muscle power. It is often not dramatic; eye movements may, in particular, be difficult.)
- EMG – there is a characteristic decrement in the evoked muscle action potential following stimulation of the motor nerve.
- CXR – may show a mediastinal mass.
- CT mediastinum – necessary in all cases to look for a thymic mass.

Management

- Pyridostigmine, an anticholinesterase, because of its sustained duration of action, is the drug of choice.
- Atropine can be given to combat the muscarinic side-effects.
- An overdose of pyridostigmine can cause severe weakness – cholinergic crisis. This may be indistinguishable from myasthenia itself. If there is this uncertainty a test dose of Tensilon can be given, with an anaesthetist and resuscitation equipment standing by.
- Pyridostigmine does not alter the natural history of the disease.
- Thymectomy is likely to benefit all patients, especially those under 40 years of age and those who have had the disease for <10 years. Following thymectomy, 60% of non-thymoma cases improve. Thymomas require surgical excision as they may be malignant; however, the myasthenia tends not to improve.
- Immunosuppression with corticosteroids or azathioprine may offer an improvement in 70% of patients who show an incomplete response to anticholinesterase.
- Plasmapheresis – to remove the circulating antibody, can be tried in emergencies. The onset of respiratory difficulty in a patient with myasthenia can rapidly become an emergency, and the facility to intubate and ventilate should be available.

11. FACIAL PALSY

Points in the examination

- The facial muscles are supplied by the facial nerve. The loss of the nasolabial fold confirms a facial palsy. However, if deepened compared to the normal side, this may signify a longstanding weakness.

The four main patterns and their aetiology

1. Unilateral weakness of all the facial muscles except the frontalis and orbicularis oris:
    - No loss of tone in the muscles, thus no sagging
    - Look for an ipsilateral limb weakness
  - Stroke or tumour – the former being by far the commonest.

2. Unilateral weakness of all facial muscles:
    - Sagging of the face with loss of tone in the muscles
    - Bell's phenomenon is seen
    - Ipsilateral loss of taste on the anterior two-thirds of the tongue
    - Ipsilateral hyperacusis
    - Look for evidence of corneal damage, conjunctivitis or a lateral tarsorrhaphy
    - Look in the external auditory meatus and at the palate for the lesions of geniculate herpes zoster (they may be seen anywhere on the head); vertigo, tinnitus or deafness may be found
    - Associated cranial nerve lesions
    - Is there evidence of aberrant reinnervation (indicating a longstanding lesion)? When they blink does the corner of the mouth twitch? When they smile does the ipsilateral eye close?
    - Lesions dissociated in space, e.g. optic atrophy, relative afferent pupillary defect, an internuclear ophthalmoplegia (INO) or ataxia
  - Bell's palsy is by far the commonest cause – other causes are rare but include:
    - Ramsay Hunt syndrome
    - Brainstem disease, e.g. multiple sclerosis (the long intrapontine course from the nucleus makes the nerve vulnerable to demyelination) and, rarely, vascular lesions – Millard–Gubler syndrome (VIth and VIIth nerve palsy and

contralateral hemiplegia), Foville syndrome (as above with conjugate gaze palsy towards the lesion)
- Mononeuropathy – of any cause, commonly diabetes or sarcoid
- Compression in the cerebellopontine angle (CPA), e.g. acoustic neuroma or meningioma (Vth, VIth, VIIth and VIIIth nerve compression).

3. Bilateral facial weakness:
    - Very easy to miss, but the patient has an expressionless face
    - Bell's phenomenon if LMN
- Acutely, it is usually due to Guillain–Barré syndrome with generalised weakness and areflexia; other causes include:
    - Sarcoid (parotid swelling and pyrexia)
    - Neuromuscular disease – facioscapulohumeral dystrophy, dystrophia myotonica or myasthenia gravis
    - Parkinson's disease – akinesia rather than weakness
    - Bilateral UMN lesions in multilacular states (pseudobulbar palsy) with a brisk jaw jerk and exaggerated involuntary movements or expressions.

4. Weakness of one or two muscles unilaterally:
    - Look for parotid enlargement or a surgical scar over the parotid or, very rarely, leprosy or an overlying skin cancer
- It is usually due to aberrant reinnervation after Bell's palsy or damage to the terminal branches of the nerve, e.g. parotid tumours, trauma, leprosy or skin cancer.

Symptoms

- Sagging or weakness of the affected side occurs.
- Dysarthria and difficulty chewing – food collects between the teeth and the gum (the muscles of mastication are, of course, intact).
- Slight alteration in sensation over the affected face – in Bell's palsy this can be ignored as long as sensation is objectively intact, including the afferent limb of the corneal reflex.
- Lacrimation may be excessive as the punctum of the lacrimal duct becomes separated from the conjunctiva. The volume of tears is, however, reduced in Bell's palsy as the parasympathetic fibres in the greater superficial petrosal nerve are interrupted.
- Deafness may be noted in patients with tumours of the CPA, the weakness and sensory loss being slight.

Investigations

- None necessary for the diagnosis of Bell's palsy
- Electrodiagnostic studies – done at 1–2 weeks after the onset can demonstrate axonal degeneration in up to 15% of those with a total paralysis
- CT brain – in UMN lesions where stroke is likely
- MRI – cerebellopontine angle tumour, demyelination or brainstem stroke
- Ultrasound then MRI – parotid tumours
- Serum ACE and ESR – sarcoidosis
- Acetylcholine receptor antibodies – if myasthenia suspected

Management

- Bell's palsy – if the paralysis is incomplete or the weakness is mild then a localised conduction block in the facial canal is likely. Provided this does not progress to more severe weakness, recovery is usually complete within a few weeks. Axonal degeneration must recover by Wallerian regeneration; thus it can take many months:
  - Corticosteroids may be of benefit, although prospective clinical trials have been inconclusive
  - Lateral tarsorrhaphy may be necessary to protect the cornea if eye closure is incomplete
  - Prostheses to elevate the angle of the mouth to reduce facial deformity may be helpful for patients with severe paralysis
  - Anastomosis of the XIth to the VIIth nerve is occasionally tried, but this must not be contemplated until adequate time for regeneration has passed – at least 9 months.
- Ramsay Hunt syndrome – aciclovir 800 mg 5 times/day for 7 days reduces symptoms. Add prednisolone 1 mg/kg, reducing over 3 weeks, for those over 60 years of age to reduce post-herpetic neuralgia. The prognosis is less favourable than for Bell's palsy.
- Stroke and tumours need investigation and treatment along standard lines.

12. PTOSIS

This patient...

Please examine this patient.

Points in the examination/aetiology

Bilateral ptosis

- Myotonic dystrophy – with frontal balding, furrowed brow, haggard face, thin neck and myotonia (see p. 252)
- Myasthenia gravis – furrowed brow, fatiguability, diplopia on sustained gaze (see p. 257)
- Ocular myopathy – ophthalmoplegia, facial/neck weakness, furrowed brow
- Bilateral Horner's syndrome – with intrinsic cord lesions, e.g. syringomyelia
- Syphilis – Argyll Robertson pupils

Unilateral ptosis

- Complete IIIn palsy – complete ptosis, pupil large, eye looking down and out (divergent strabismus), diplopia on adduction. The other eye is usually normal. The pupil is spared in a medial IIIrd nerve palsy – usually due to diabetes mellitus.
- Partial IIIn palsy – partial ptosis with a large pupil on the affected side. If there is proptosis of the eye suspect an orbital tumour or vascular anomaly – listen for a bruit over the eye.
- Horner's syndrome – partial ptosis, pupil small on affected side. Pupils normally reactive and movements normal. May have anhidrosis on the affected side. Good lateralising but poor localising sign, thus look for:
  - Loss of the corneal reflex ipsilaterally – orbital or retro-orbital tumour
  - Weakness, wasting and hypo/areflexia in the ipsilateral upper limb – avulsion injury to the brachial plexus or Pancoast's tumour
  - Ipsilateral loss of pain and temperature sensation – brainstem lesion (bilateral disease may be present).
- NB. Any cause of bilateral ptosis may cause unilateral disease.

Symptoms

The pattern of symptoms reflects the cause (see the appropriate sections).

Investigations

- Glucose – diabetes mellitus
- ESR/CRP – other causes of mononeuritis – rheumatoid arthritis, SLE, PAN, Wegener's granulomatosis, sarcoid
- Anticholinesterase antibodies – 100% specific and 90% sensitive for myasthenia
- CXR – apical malignancy or cervical rib
- Syphilis serology
- MRI – in the investigation of IIIn palsy of uncertain aetiology
- Electromyography

Management

- Dependent on the cause.

Points of interest

- If Horner's syndrome has been present from birth the iris remains blue while the other may become brown – heterochromia.
- Mechanical ptosis may occur in an elderly patient due to dehiscence of the levator palpebrae superioris; there are no associated signs.
- In a complete IIIrd nerve palsy there may be mild proptosis when the patient sits up due to loss of tone in the extraocular muscles; it disappears on lying down.

13. NYSTAGMUS

Points in the examination

- The direction of nystagmus is defined by the direction of the fast phase. However, the slow phase is the pathological component; the fast phase is the correction.
- Attempting to lateralise the location of the lesion on the basis of the nystagmus alone is folly.
- Short-term horizontal nystagmus at the extremes of lateral gaze is physiological.
- Horizontal nystagmus which only occurs on looking laterally – this is either due to a central or peripheral lesion:
  - In a peripheral lesion the direction of the fast phase is away from the lesion
  - In a central lesion the direction of the fast phase is towards the lesion.

Aetiology

- Peripheral lesions – caused by a process involving connections between the labyrinth and the vestibular apparatus.
- Central lesions – caused by brainstem or cerebellar pathology. The likely pathology is either demyelination, stroke or tumour and, rarely, hereditary causes, e.g. Friedreich's ataxia (see p. 244):
  - Examine the external auditory meatus and drum, and look for scars, e.g. over the mastoid process
  - Test hearing grossly: if abnormal go on to perform Weber's and Rinné's tests. If doubt remains, proceed to a pure-tone audiogram
  - Examine for hemiparesis, cerebellar signs and optic nerve damage, considering demyelination, strokes and tumours
  - Look for evidence of a cerebellopontine angle tumour – this involves the Vth, VIth, VIIth and VIIIth nerves. The earliest sign is the loss of the corneal reflex – the afferent limb is the Vth nerve and efferent the VIIth nerve; thus the contralateral corneal reflex results in bilateral lid closure. Later, facial sensation is impaired, then facial weakness occurs. Deafness is an early feature but may need an audiogram to demonstrate.

- Prolonged horizontal nystagmus on lateral gaze bilaterally – commonly drugs (e.g. phenytoin, barbiturates and benzodiazepines) and alcohol. All these drugs may also cause vertical nystagmus. It may occasionally result from the brainstem and cerebellar lesions mentioned above, e.g. MS affecting both cerebellar hemispheres.
- Vertical nystagmus:
  - Upbeat – Wernicke's encephalopathy, MS, brainstem tumours
  - Downbeat – tumours at the foramen magnum.
- Ataxic nystagmus – closely allied to INO (see p. 207).
- Pendular – no fast phase. Congenital or retinal pathology (e.g. loss of macular vision).
- Converging – due to lesions involving the midbrain centre for convergence and vertical gaze located at the pretectal plate in the roof of the midbrain (Parinaud's syndrome). Patients cannot look up and convergent nystagmus occurs; pupillary responses and convergence can all be abnormal but accommodation is unaffected. They have a tendency to fall backwards. Causes include pinealoma, hydrocephalus and stroke.

Symptoms

- Oscillopsia.
- Dizziness and vertigo may be associated with vestibular or central abnormalities.

Investigations

- Pure-tone audiogram and caloric tests for peripheral VIIIn function
- MRI – if lesions at the CPA, brainstem, cerebellum or demyelination suspected
- Phenytoin level
- Blood alcohol, γ-GT, LFT
- Red cell transketolase (Wernicke's encephalopathy)

Management

- Dependent on the cause.

STATION 4

The Communication Skills and Ethics' Examination

Approach to the Communication Skills' Station

The ability to communicate effectively with a colleague, patient or relative is a fundamental tenet of practising medicine and the communication skills' station in PACES tests one's ability to do this. As with history-taking, many candidates feel they are already skilled in this aspect and do not prepare adequately for this station. The aims of the station are to explore the candidate's ability to engage in a two-way form of communication, to listen and respond to patients' concerns and to impart upsetting news in a sensitive and empathic manner. The examination scenarios often require the candidate to have some knowledge of both medical ethics and medicolegal issues pertaining to everyday clinical practice. The following section discusses these issues and offers some guidelines as to how to break bad news and to communicate sensitive matters, before discussing 20 scenarios. These will cover the vast majority of clinical situations that a candidate may be expected to deal with.

BACKGROUND

The communication skills and ethics station in PACES is about imparting information on a subject in a clear and coherent manner. It aims to assess the candidate's ability to guide and organise the interview with the patient. Interaction with the patient is essential. It is not a test of medical knowledge. It is more important to put the patient at ease, establish a good rapport and understand their anxieties and needs, rather than devising a brilliant management plan.

In this part of the exam it is much more important for candidates to understand the needs of a patient, and to build a good rapport with them, than to know the thirteenth cause of diabetes insipidus. Coming across as sensible and level-headed is more important than knowing all the answers to the questions. This section is designed to weed out candidates who, despite being extremely bright, are poor at discussing sensitive issues at the appropriate level.

By the time candidates arrive at this stage of the exam they have already proved in the written part to have sufficient knowledge of the subject matter. The importance of this station is to demonstrate competence in translating this knowledge to the clinical setting. It is exactly this that makes the Communication Skills' Station such a valid and discriminatory part of PACES.

The paternalistic approach to consultation is currently out of step with society. Approaching consultations from a mutual position of strength may be an ideal; however, one cannot forget that at times succinct advice and information must be given, perhaps not even in a sympathetic manner. The goal of the truly complete doctor is to 'be all things to all men', which is clearly unattainable.

APPROACH TO THE STATION

The Communication Skills' Station of the exam is split into three parts.

PART 1

5 minutes outside the room to read the provided instructions

Read the instructions very carefully.

Establish the key issues, which must be conveyed, and the take-home messages from the consultation which the patient must have understood. Patients rarely remember more than two or three pieces of information from a consultation.

Only after the consultation has started, and the expectations and knowledge of the patient established, can the candidate work out the most appropriate way of conveying these messages.

The written scenario will contain the information about the problems surrounding the case. Further history-taking questions should be unnecessary – the information given should be taken as complete.

Consider the medical, legal and ethical issues surrounding the patient. These are areas of specific concern to the examiners and marking is geared towards the candidate's ability to discuss them.

Consider the important issues of the consultation, but do not set the direction in stone – the direction depends entirely on the interactions of the patient and doctor. It is important to remain flexible.

PART 2

The interview – 15 minutes (including 1 minute to gather one's thoughts at the end)

Introduction

- Introduce yourself and explain your role.
- Ensure the positioning of the furniture is correct.
- Try to put the patient at ease.

The discussion

- Candidates should try to strike a balance between appearing knowledgeable and confident, as well as considerate and approachable.
- The consultation should be pitched at the correct level for the patient.
- Allow the patient to speak openly and freely, but be prepared to direct the consultation.
- Establish the expectations and knowledge of the patient with open questions, e.g.: 'We have not met before; you have come today to talk about your kidney problems; what do you understand about what is going on?'
- Consider why has this particular patient presented to you at this time?
- Explain to the patient the options from here, and the implication of these options.
- Try to give the patient choices rather than instructions.
- Allow pauses for the patient to digest information.
- If a part of the consultation has gone badly it is reasonable to go over that specific part again. Under these circumstances stop and ask, 'I have said quite a lot, do you want me to go over some of it again before we move on?' There is little point in moving from one area to another, covering all the information required, if the patient is taking none of it in. It is far better for the patient to have secured one or two key facts rather than a huge jumbled blur of information.
- While you are following instructions and working to an agenda, to fail to do anything well in the hope of covering everything (albeit poorly) will result in failure.

- Under certain circumstances, it is reasonable not to cover all the possible information from the instructions. For instance, there may be a lack of time (rushing through lists of information is not good communication), or the patient may have heard enough, e.g.: 'I would rather come back with my family before we discuss this more.'
- It may be inappropriate to cover all the information once the patient's expectations have been assessed, e.g. discussing resuscitation in a patient who is clearly in shock after receiving bad news.
- If all the information has not been covered, do not panic; tell the examiners why this has happened during your discussion with them. If you can defend your conduct in a professional manner, success is likely.

Before finishing

- Summarise the consultation.
- Agree a management plan for the future.
- Ask if they want anything repeated or if they have any questions.
- Ask if there are any important issues that have not been covered.
- Arrange another appointment if necessary.

Gathering thoughts – 1 minute

- Order the information in your mind.
- Anticipate the likely discussion points with the examiners.

PART 3

5 minutes of discussion with the examiners

The following issues are likely to be discussed:
- How do you think it went; good areas and bad areas?
- What could be done differently?
- What do you think the patient has understood?
- How you would approach follow-up consultations?
- Which areas were not covered?
- Have the needs of the patient been met?
- What are the legal and ethical issues surrounding the case?
- What would the further management and follow-up arrangements be?

The candidate should remain flexible during this period with the examiners. No two consultations are the same, and sometimes one approach works better than another. It is reasonable to say that with hindsight you would have done things differently, and in follow-up consultations would readdress areas that were covered badly or not covered at all.

Once again, detailed medical information is not required; the examiners are much more interested in the following:

- Was the patient put at ease?
- Were the questions open and at the right level?
- Did the candidate strike a balance between appearing confident, knowledgeable and approachable?
- Were the key issues discussed openly?
- How did the candidate handle sensitive issues?
- Were the key messages conveyed well?

BREAKING BAD NEWS

Individuals are influenced by social, cultural and religious beliefs. Therefore there is no single approach to breaking bad news that will satisfy all patients. However, a uniform, well-practised method, with flexibility dependent on the situation, can calm these choppy waters.

In reality, doctors will often have known the patient for some time, making the consultation easier. For PACES this is not practical.

Classic worst-case scenario:
Doctor: 'So how long have you been on this treatment for your prostate cancer?'
Patient: 'No-one's told me I've got cancer.'
Never assume anything.

The 8 steps to breaking bad news:

1. The right information
2. The right place
3. The right people – ask the patient if there is anyone they would like present
4. Introduction
5. Establish what the patient knows
6. Informing the patient
7. Questions
8. Finishing

The key to breaking bad news is in the preparation.

1. The right information

- Check all the information yourself, e.g. the histology/CT scans – do not rely on hearsay.
- Ensure all the information needed is present before starting to break the news.
- Speak to the nursing staff looking after the patient to ascertain what the patient knows and expects.
- After breaking bad news the patient is likely to ask about future management plans; doctors should have management options for the patient before starting to break bad news.

2. The right place

- Choose a quiet location where a conversation cannot be overheard; turn off your bleep, pager or mobile phone.
- Do not conduct the consultation across a desk, or an intervening barrier.
- Do not appear rushed, but conduct the consultation in a calm, reassuring and sympathetic manner.

3. The right people

- Ask the nursing staff involved with the care of the patient if they would like to be present. They may have had time to form a useful relationship with the patient.
- If the patient has visitors it is often best to come back later.
- Before starting, ask the patient if they would like anyone present, e.g. friend or family member(s). It is often helpful for them to have a close friend or relative present to offer emotional support. Under stressful situations the patient often retains very little of the information given.

4. Introduction

- Introduce yourself to the patient.
- Explain your role in the medical team.
- Maintain good eye contact.

5. Establish what the patient knows

- 'What have the other doctors told you about what is going on?'
- 'Do you understand why we have been doing these tests or suspect what might be wrong?'

Patients tend to fall in to two main groups – those who have a pretty good idea of what is going on and those who do not.

6. Informing the patient

Patients with insight:
- These patients will usually say something like – 'Yes, we were looking for multiple sclerosis, what do the tests show?' – this is the easy group.
- Tell the patient in broad terms – details are often forgotten in this stressful situation.
- Avoid medical jargon.
- Talk slowly and clearly.
- Use pauses to allow the patient to react.
- Never lie or guess.
- Ask if there is anything they didn't understand or want repeated.
- Keep the tone sympathetic but positive.
- Summarise what has been said.

Patients without insight:
- This is a more difficult consultation, and is the scenario where most of the problems arise.
- The key is to give warning shots – e.g. 'Your condition appears to be quite serious' or 'Some of the test results are not good' – with small nuggets of information, allowing sufficient pauses for the patient to comprehend and respond; then ask if they want more information.
- If so, continue with another small amount of information and ask if they want to know more.
- If not, explain that you will come back later, and if they think of any questions to ask them then.
- Suggest it might be helpful to have members of the family present for support.
- Often the patient is just not fully prepared in themselves at that point and the consultation is often easier on the second occasion.
- The second consultation should start where the previous conversation left off, recapping on ground already covered.

It must be stressed that this is by no means the only way to break bad news. Any well-rehearsed and successful method is clearly acceptable.

7. Questions

Before leaving, ask the patient if there is anything they would like to ask.
The most common question is, 'How long have I got?'
- Prognosis:
  - It is impossible to convey all the information in one sitting, and
    discussing prognosis is usually best left for follow-up
    consultations. Prognosis varies enormously from one individual
    to another and depends on the response to treatment. However,
    it is perhaps prudent to avoid prognostication at all costs as it is so
    fraught with uncertainty.
- If asked a question directly and you do not know the answer, never
  lie or guess. Explain that you will attempt to find the correct answer
  for the next consultation or later that day, as appropriate.
  - If the doctor knows the prognosis, response to treatment and
    outcomes of the disease:
    - 'No one knows what will happen in the future, and so I do not
      like to give exact figures. Everybody is different and some
      people do much better than others. However, we should
      probably think in terms of months rather than years, but once
      again no one really knows.' (If the prognosis is months.)
- The next question often relates to cure: 'But there is a chance I will
  get better isn't there doctor?' The patient is now looking for hope,
  and is it important not to quash this completely. However, it is
  essential to prepare the patient for the inevitable in a delicate
  manner.
  - A useful phrase to introduce the concept of a terminal illness is:
    'I do not think this disease will ever go away completely.
    Allowing time for patient reaction is important.
- Do not necessarily tell terminally ill patients to give up smoking or
  drinking. The horse has already bolted.

8. Finishing

- Summarise what has been said.
- Ask if they have understood everything.
- Ask if they want anything repeated.
- Ask if they have any further questions.
- Give a contact number.
- Make a follow-up appointment.

Difficult situations

The daughter knows her mother has cancer but does not want you to tell her mother

Legal and ethical issues

- The duty of care is to the mother.
- The daughter should not have found out – although there is nothing you can do about that now.
- The daughter knows the patient much better than you do, and might be right.
- Ultimately, both the patient and healthcare team may rely on the daughter to support the patient; a breakdown in the relationship with her would therefore be a disaster.

Approach to the daughter

- As above, check the information and speak to the other carers looking after the patient.
- Take the daughter to a quiet room.
- Ask how she knows the diagnosis.
- Ask how she knows how her mother does not know.
- Ask why she does not want her mother to know.
- Explain that you appreciate that she knows her mother much better than the doctors. However, having seen this situation many times before, telling the mother the truth is usually what she wants and is best in the long term.
    - 'Deep down, most people know when there is something seriously wrong, and finding out can be a relief.'
- Explain to the daughter that you need to be sure that her mother does not want to know her diagnosis.
- Explain that you will talk to the mother and give her a small amount of information, and will answer questions truthfully leading from that.
    - 'If she does not want to know I will not tell her.'
    - Follow the 'Informing patients with no insight' approach (see p. 275), giving only small amounts of information at a time.

Patients who have been previously misinformed before your consultation

Common examples:
- Patients who have been told curative treatment is available, when it is not, or
- That surgery will be next week, when the waiting list is much longer
- Patients given the wrong diagnosis/prognosis/treatment, or
- Informed that results will be available, when they are not

What to say:
- Check the information you have is correct.
- Explain that the previous information is not correct.
- Explain that whatever has happened in the past is now out of your control.
- Explain that the key now is to look to the best treatment for the future.
- Make an attempt to find out why things went wrong in the past.
- Offer the patient a second opinion if they want one.
- The chances are that the patient will be angry with the medical profession as a whole, and you are the person available to vent their anger on.
- Even though you are not responsible, an apology may well be appropriate.
- An overdefensive or aggressive approach from you will be counterproductive.
- The best approach is to weather the storm and remain calm. Once the patient has expressed their opinion, suggest you will find out what went wrong and to stop it happening again, but that now you must try to focus on the future and the current medical problems.

Admitting your own mistakes to patients and other doctors

It is very easy to make a mistake in medicine; admitting to them is slightly more difficult.

The key is honesty with patients and colleagues at an early stage. Any attempt to lie or cover up may backfire in a most dramatic fashion.

Approach to the patient:
- Most patients understand that nobody is perfect, and that that applies to doctors too!
- Be honest and apologetic.
- Tell the patient at the first available opportunity.
- Explain what the plan was and what went wrong.

- Explain what the options are in the future (including seeking a second opinion).
- Explain how you will try to prevent the same mistake happening again.
- Listen carefully to what the patient has to say.

Surprisingly, most patients will take the issue no further, providing they feel that the explanation is satisfactory and that the individuals are truly apologetic.

Most formal complaints or litigation issues are due to a breakdown in the doctor–patient relationship and poor communication skills, rather than the mistake itself.

Ethical and Legal Issues in Medicine

INTRODUCTION

Although communication skills are of paramount importance in a patient consultation, it is also essential that doctors are aware of the legal and ethical issues surrounding a few difficult issues. It is impossible for a candidate to discuss these issues if they are unaware of the rules that govern them. It should be remembered that, in real life, making difficult legal or ethical decisions alone is usually a mistake; involving other professionals makes the process easier and gives a more balanced opinion. Medical defence organisations offer legal and ethical advice 24 hours a day to members.

Although, one's cultural background and personal beliefs influence one's approach to a patient when discussing ethical issues, it is vitally important to be able to put these to one side and to respect an individual's legal rights. These rights have changed over the years, but in the UK are currently defined by the Human Rights Act of 1998. There are numerous articles within this convention, including the right to liberty and the right to respect a private life. It is also clearly stated that it is unlawful for a public authority, such as the NHS, to contravene this convention.

CONSENT

The philosophy that 'Doctor knows best' is a thoroughly outdated way to practise medicine; patients have the right to self-determination and, after an informed two-way discussion, can refuse any suggested treatment except where covered by the Mental Health Act (1983).

In order to obtain consent, an individual must be deemed competent to understand and retain the information, using it to reach a reasonable decision. This decision requires a patient to be accurately informed as to the nature and risks of the planned procedure. Legally, any non-consensual contact is the tort of battery.

How much does the patient need to know?

In the UK, patients do not necessarily have to be informed of every side-effect or risk from a specific treatment. Patients should understand 'in broad terms' the nature of the events; doctors can withhold information from a patient on the grounds of 'therapeutic privilege' (*Chatterton* v. *Gerson* 1981). It is not always deemed to be in the best interests of the patient to discuss extremely unlikely side-effects, as it may lead to undue anxiety and poor decision-making.

In general terms, patients should be told of all common side-effects, even if not serious; and all serious side-effects, even if rare.

Situations where consent is not possible

Unconscious patients are unable to give the necessary consent required for treatment. Under these circumstances doctors can give emergency treatment if it is in the best interests of the patient, the 'doctrine of necessity'. If relatives are available for discussion they should be informed rather than opinions canvassed. It is advisable that they remain well informed.

If mental impairment is suspected a psychiatrist must be consulted to make the diagnosis – defined as 'any disability or disorder of the mind or brain, whether permanent or temporary, which results in impairment or disturbance of mental function' – the patient is unable to give consent. The legal situation and the medical management of these patients may be complicated. Guardians and relatives have no legal rights. In these situations, medical staff may be required to make decisions which are deemed to be in the best interests of the patient, without obtaining informed consent. These decisions should be consistent with a reasonable body of medical opinion – this is known as the Bolam test (*Bolam* v. *Friern HMC* 1957). Reform to the law on mental capacity is underway. A general authority will act for the personal welfare of any individual who lacks the ability to give consent for ongoing treatment, thus relieving the burden on medical staff.

Detainment of patients against their will under the 1983 Mental Health Act is aimed at controlling patients who are a danger either to themselves or to others due to temporary or permanent mental illness. They can be detained/restrained for varying periods, depending on the clause of the Act, and can be given treatment, but only for their mental illness, which is deemed in their best interests or the best interests of the public.

Advance directives are made prospectively in order to convey a person's wishes on specific matters in case that person is unable to give subsequent consent due to incompetence for whatever reason. They are recognised in law and must be respected, as long as they are completed by a competent, witnessed, adult. Patients should seek the help of a medical practitioner when completing an advance directive. Review of advance directives is recommended periodically.

Relatives have a legal influence with regard to giving consent in only two situations: in minors who are not 'Gillick competent' and after death (q.v.).

The Family Law Reform Act of 1969 defines a minor as below 18 years of age. However, for the purposes of medical treatment a patient achieves adult status at 16. A competent child between 16 and 18 years of age can therefore give valid consent to any surgical, medical or dental treatment, regardless of parental opinion. Where the ages of 16 and 17 years are important is in cases of mental incompetence, in which situation a parent can act for them until they become of age.

Children under the age of 16 years can give consent for medical intervention, or refuse it, if they are deemed to be of sufficient maturity and intelligence to understand the implications of the treatment. This is referred to as 'Gillick competence' (*Gillick v. West Norfolk and Wisbech AHA* 1985), e.g. prescribing the oral contraceptive pill to a 14-year-old girl without the consent of the parents is only allowed if the child has sufficient maturity to understand the implications of the treatment.

Parents must act in the best interests of their child in order to give valid consent. If it is deemed by the medical staff that this is not the case, the child can be made a ward of court and treatment given without the parents' consent. However, this should be the last course of action. Acting against the parents' wishes will usually result in a breakdown in the doctor–patient/parent relationship, and may ultimately compromise the healthcare of the individual. Often, taking time to explain the situation and building a trusting relationship with the people involved is an easier way to proceed.

CONFIDENTIALITY

In order to maintain a good patient relationship, consultations should be carried out in confidence. One must, by law, breach confidence in certain circumstances, and at other times one may breach confidence if deemed in the best interests of the patient. The latter situations are more common and potentially more difficult from an ethical perspective. Contrary to a widespread belief by both medical practitioners and the public, relatives, other than the parents of a child, are not privy to any medical details of an individual in any circumstance. However, in order to act in the best interests of a patient, confidence must occasionally be broken. For example, if a patient is unconscious it may be in their best interests to break confidence, not only to obtain more information, but also to relieve the anxiety of the relatives. It may become impossible to manage a patient effectively without allowing the relatives on board. Striking a balance between keeping relatives happy and obtaining as much information as possible, whilst respecting the rights of an individual, is difficult.

Confidentiality is often breached in hospital for the purposes of cross-specialty care. Consent for this is generally assumed by patients and doctors alike. However, this is implied consent and there may be occasions where specific consent must be sought.

Situations where confidentiality must be broken

- Notifiable diseases (e.g. TB, plague and food poisoning)
- Under Section 18 of the Prevention of Terrorism Act 1989
- If a warrant from a circuit judge has been obtained
- Individuals who have been involved in a road traffic accident. A doctor who suspects a patient has been involved in a road traffic accident is under a duty to give information to the police, but only in order to identify the driver (*Hunter* v. *Mann* 1974)

Situations where confidentiality can be broken

- Where one is acting in the best interests of the patient (only if unconscious, or confused)
- Acting in the best interests of society:
  - For example, AIDS is not a notifiable disease and individuals have the right to confidentiality. While the patient should be strongly encouraged to inform others at risk, they do not have to do so. However, in exceptional circumstances, where it is considered to be of benefit to society, disclosing information can be done without the express consent of the patient, i.e. to prevent potential harm to other individuals

- While the Courts in England and Wales are reluctant to make person 'A' liable for the crimes of person 'B', the extent of a doctor's duty to a third party in England and Wales would appear to be that a doctor must not ignore the risk to others created by a patient, but weigh up one's duty to society against one's duty to an individual

Situations where confidentiality should not be broken

In cases of sexually transmitted disease and abortions confidentiality must be maintained.

This respect of confidentiality also applies after the patient has died. 'I will respect the secrets which are confided in me even after the patient has died' – Declaration of Geneva (as amended in Sydney 1968).

NEGLIGENCE

Three separate issues are involved in demonstrating negligence in the UK.

- A duty of care between the doctor and patient must be established. For example, a doctor is not obliged to help someone in distress on the street because no duty of care has been established.
- A breach of this duty of care must be demonstrated. The patient must show that the treatment was not in accordance with a reasonable body of medical opinion (Bolam test, q.v.). This is an area of controversy and allows doctors to self-regulate. In the light of recent events in the UK and subsequent press interest, self-regulation may become a thing of the past. The future points towards an independent body, with members of the public involved in regulation of the medical profession.
- This breach of duty of care caused harm. The claim should be brought within 3 years of the action occurring, unless under exceptional circumstances.

In the UK, financial reward for a successful claim is aimed at compensating the individual or family rather than punishing the guilty parties. The Woolf reforms (2000) made the process of a claim quicker and easier. Most cases should be settled out of court, and a claim should be acknowledged within 21 days.

HOSPITAL NOTES

Patients have the right to see their medical notes and computer records, which are subject to the Data Protection Act 1998. If a patient asks to review their notes it should be done with a member of the medical team, to explain medical terms.

Individuals not directly involved in the health of the patient must obtain consent to see the medical records.

LIFE AND DEATH

From a legal point of view, life ends when brainstem death occurs. There are a series of tests which must be carried out to confirm this. It is possible for respiration to be supported artificially, even once brainstem death has occurred (i.e. ventilation). Withdrawing artificial support once a diagnosis of brainstem death has been made requires a series of steps, detailed below. These patients are often candidates for organ donation.

Diagnosing brainstem death

- Deep coma with absent respiration
- Absence of hypoxia, hypothermia, hypoglycaemia, acidosis, abnormal biochemistry and sedative drugs

Tests

These include:
- Fixed dilated pupils, absent corneal response and vestibulo-ocular reflex
- No gag reflex or motor response in the cranial nerves
- No respiratory effort on stopping the ventilator and allowing the $PaCO_2$ to rise to 6.7 kPa

The tests should be performed by a consultant or his deputy in the presence of another doctor. The tests should be repeated after at least a 24-hour interval.

In the USA, an EEG is required to confirm brain death.

Persistent Vegetative State (PVS)

Patients whose brainstem function persists despite loss of cortical function, are described as having a persistent vegetative state. Their quality of life is at best uncertain, and their life depends on artificial feeding. However, it is only possible to withdraw this feeding via a court order. The test case for this was that of Tony Bland, who was diagnosed with PVS after the Hillsborough disaster. The test case was heard by the House of Lords – the doctors and relatives involved felt feeding should be stopped, their Lordships agreed and feeding was subsequently withdrawn.

Euthanasia

Competent patients have the right to refuse any active treatment that may prolong their life. However, euthanasia – the process of accelerating death by active intervention artificially – is viewed in a different way. Currently, active euthanasia is illegal in the UK. Test cases have been unsuccessful in altering this premise (R. v. Cox 1992). The only country to allow active euthanasia is Holland, but it is subject to strict guidelines. The USA remains against active euthanasia.

Under present legislation in the UK, doctors performing an intervention to terminate life are guilty of manslaughter, despite the wishes of the patient.

Whether accelerating the death of a terminally ill individual is in their best interests is open to debate. The termination of life contradicts many firmly held religious beliefs across a wide spectrum of faiths and results in heated debate. These decisions on euthanasia should be made by society as a whole and reflected in legislation. Doctors must act within the law and may need to compromise their own personal beliefs.

Doctors can administer symptomatic treatment, which has known adverse side-effects. This is the 'principle of double effect'. A classic example is increasing doses of opiates to control the pain of terminally ill patients, but which may also hasten the process of death. From a medical point of view it would be generally accepted that the paramount objective is to alleviate suffering by relieving the pain, and that the administration of large doses of opiates is acting in the best interests of the patient. Do not take decisions of this magnitude alone, discuss with colleagues, nurses, the patient and their family as appropriate, and carefully document all decisions and discussions in the medical notes.

Once a duty of care is established then doctors must act in the best interests of the patient. Omitting treatment that may prolong suffering does not necessarily break that duty of care, e.g. not prescribing antibiotics for infections. This omission of treatment is called 'passive euthanasia'. Any ongoing treatment that is futile should be stopped in terminally ill patients. Administering an ineffective treatment with symptomatic side-effects is not in the best interests of the patient as the side-effects outweigh the benefits.

RESUSCITATION

Discussing resuscitation status with the patient is strongly encouraged and this should be done wherever possible or reasonable, a view supported by the GMC. However, common sense governs the timing of such a discussion, e.g. it is probably inappropriate with relatively fit young patients where it would lead to unnecessary anxiety. Patients remain for resuscitation until a decision has been made. Resuscitation should be attempted if there is any uncertainty about the decision of the patient or nature of the disease. If a competent patient does not wish to be resuscitated this should be respected.

Resuscitation should not be performed if it is deemed futile, or not in the best interests of the patient. Resuscitation can be an inhumane act under certain circumstances. If a decision not to resuscitate has been made, it should be clearly documented in the medical notes.

If the patient is unconscious, discussion with the relatives may give an impression of what the patient might have wanted. A doctor does not consult relatives for their opinion on the right course of action, although this should be respected. The opinion or wishes of relatives regarding resuscitation has no legal standing.

GYNAECOLOGICAL ISSUES

Infertility treatment and abortion are areas of intense legal and ethical debate. For the purposes of PACES we will not dwell on them, as they are unlikely to be featured in the exam. However, having some general knowledge is reasonable. The 1967 Abortion Act states that a pregnancy can be terminated if the pregnancy has not exceeded 24 weeks, providing continuing the pregnancy poses a risk to the mental or physical health of the mother, or existing children.

It can be carried out up to term if the baby is physically or mentally handicapped. Termination of pregnancy remains illegal in Ireland and the sanctity of life is one of the cornerstones of the Roman Catholic Church.

OWNERSHIP OF BODY PARTS

While the Nuffield Report 1995 states that any consent to medical intervention implies tissue removed is regarded as abandoned, this is currently too simplistic. Recent well-publicised events have led to a change in opinion and it is now widely accepted that specific consent is required for organ/tissue retention. This issue is an area of intense debate and legislation is likely to be forthcoming.

ORGAN DONATION

If the patient expressed a wish to donate organs after death this should be respected. However, relatives must give consent for donation and must be consulted; they can refuse donation even if the deceased's wishes were well known. After death, the next of kin have lawful possession of the body. If someone dies and there are no next of kin then the hospital has possession. Once transplantation has taken place the organs are the possession of the recipient.

Although advance directives are legal documents, organ donor cards are not; they only give an impression of what the deceased wished at the time of completion.

- Organ donation from a live donor must not be detrimental to the health of that individual.
- The donor need not be an adult, e.g. matched related bone marrow donation.
- Once donated, the organ is the possession of the recipient.
- Organs cannot be legally bought or sold in the UK. If a donation is to take place between two unrelated individuals it must be referred to the Unrelated Live Transplantation Authority.

RESEARCH

Research projects should only commence after the approval of a research and ethics committee has been given. It is unlawful to carry out research on patients who are unable to give consent. Samples taken cannot be used for research retrospectively if consent was not given specifically when the samples were taken, although these samples are not deemed the property of the patient.

ALLOCATION OF RESOURCES

Individuals would like to be given the most appropriate healthcare at the most favourable time. However, limited resources inevitably results in rationing, and society decides what it can and cannot afford. Care is often delivered from a waiting list, with emergency intervention taking priority. In the UK, The National Institute of Clinical Excellence (NICE) assesses treatments for their clinical and financial effectiveness. This method of allocation is known as a 'utilitarian approach', which roughly translates as aiming to provide the greatest utility for the greatest number of people.

Deontological theory views ethical issues from a different angle, and is based on selecting the optimal treatment for the individual regardless of resources. These two theories often contradict one another. For example, an expensive drug may not be approved by NICE, despite showing a benefit to certain patient groups. Under these circumstances, NICE would argue that the cost outweighs the benefit to society as a whole, and the resources may be better placed elsewhere.

Communication Skills and Ethics' Scenarios

The following 20 examples demonstrate the wide range of different scenarios a candidate may face. The discussion which follows should be seen only as a guide rather than 'the correct answer', pointing candidates in the correct direction. The consultation may progress in many different directions and each scenario gives the opposite extremes a candidate might face. Most consultations will fall somewhere between these extremes.

1.

You are the neurology SHO. A 24-year-old fashion model was diagnosed as having 'grand mal' epilepsy 6 months ago, but has failed to attend for follow-up appointments. In the last few weeks she has had several fits. She has an extremely busy social lifestyle and claims that she 'needs to drive a car' because of her work and social commitments, which she is still doing. She attends many late-night parties and drinks 20–30 units of alcohol a week; she also takes recreational drugs. Whilst she is keen for any help to prevent her fits, she is very unwilling to take regular medication.

Please discuss the management of her epilepsy.

Preliminary thoughts

- Effects of alcohol/cocaine on epilepsy
- Legal issues regarding patient confidentiality vs. informing the DVLA (see p. 283)
- Medical treatment options

Goals of the consultation

- Avoid scaring her off and maintain her trust.
- Ensure she stops driving and informs the DVLA; if she does not, you will have to.
- For her to understand that:
  - Her fits will continue or get worse if she does not seek help
  - The fits may stop if she changes her lifestyle and seeks help.

Key points in the consultation

- Introduce yourself and put the patient at ease.
- Establish the patient's expectations/fears – why has she turned up today?
- Establish this patient's level of understanding of her diagnosis, complications and possible treatment.
- Establish her knowledge of precipitating factors, including alcohol, recreational drugs, late nights and general lifestyle.
- Discuss the importance and benefits of stopping/preventing such precipitating factors.

- Maintain a balance between realistic aims and ideal aims. Is it likely that she will significantly change her behaviour?
- Discuss her need for possible medication, side-effects, drug interactions (especially with the oral contraceptive pill (OCP)).
- Impress upon her the ethical issues of continuing to drive and her responsibility to society.
- Emphasise the legal requirement for her to inform the DVLA and to stop driving (possibility of recommencing driving if fit-free for 1 year), but that you have a legal duty to inform the DVLA if, in the future, you suspect she is continuing to drive.
- Emphasise that the majority of patients are free from medication within 5 years.

Directions of the consultation

Scenario A

The patient remains adamant that her lifestyle and fits are unrelated and/or is unwilling to stop driving.

- It is important to repeatedly stress to her the seriousness of her condition and the ethical issues associated with her continuing to drive: a firm but sympathetic approach may be required.
- All discussions should be well documented in her medical notes.
- As it is important for her to maintain faith in you, some form of compromise may be appropriate. For example, stopping the recreational drugs for a week and returning to the clinic to see how things are. No compromise can be made concerning the driving.
- She should be aware that ultimately you may have to inform the DVLA.

Scenario B

She accepts the nature of her condition and agrees to modify her lifestyle, but is unwilling to stop driving.

- A more sympathetic approach should be adopted, but stressing the legal and ethical reasons to stop driving.
- She should be aware that if she goes along with the medical advice and modifies her lifestyle, there is a good chance her health will return to normal and she will be able to lead a normal life, including driving.

Finishing

- Ask her if she has any questions.
- Ensure she understands the nature of her condition.
- Make follow-up arrangements.

Discussion

The GMC and DVLA criteria for driving (Oct 2001) – see also p. 115

If a patient is suffering from a condition that may affect their driving, the onus lies with *them* to report this to the DVLA. If the patient is incapable of understanding this advice, the doctor should inform the DVLA immediately. Ultimately the DVLA is legally responsible for deciding if that patient is medically fit to drive. If the patient refuses to accept their doctor's diagnosis, the doctor should suggest a second opinion. If the patient continues to drive when considered unfit, the doctor should report this to the medical officer at the DVLA. Before discussing legal issues it is often beneficial to discuss the ethical context in which the law arises. Individuals are more likely to comply with legislation if they understand the reasoning behind it. Candidates should be aware of the current regulations regarding medical restrictions on driving (*www.dvla.gov.uk*).

2.

A 55-year-old man has returned to the gastroenterology outpatient clinic for a review of his ulcerative colitis. He has had this for more than 10 years, during which time he has had numerous courses of oral steroids for exacerbations and is on long-term azathioprine. Over the last 6 months he has had worsening diarrhoea and currently opens his bowels approximately 10 times a day. A recent colonoscopy has revealed active pancolitis. He is increasingly 'fed up' with his condition.

Please discuss his management with a view to recommending total colectomy.

Preliminary thoughts

- Long-term symptoms and complications of ulcerative colitis (UC) and prognosis:
  - Carcinoma/bowel obstruction
  - Toxic megacolon
- Risks of surgery
- Practicalities of stoma – discuss with stoma nurse
- Patient support groups
- Legal and ethical issues – competent individuals have the right of self-determination, and this must be respected (see *Consent*, p. 281)

Goals of the consultation

- The patient understands why colectomy is the most viable option.
- He is aware of the benefits and risks.
- He gains sufficient knowledge to make an informed decision, although not necessarily immediately.

Key points in the consultation

- Introduce yourself to the patient and establish rapport.
- Establish the patient's understanding and knowledge of his condition, its severity and long-term complications.
- Establish the patient's expectations (cure/incurable).
- Explain the severity of his condition and its increasing unresponsiveness to medical therapy (see *Breaking bad news*, p. 273).
- Explain the risk of colonic carcinoma and toxic megacolon in long-term active pancolitis.

- Introduce the idea of a total colectomy – discuss:
  - Benefits of symptom relief and a more normal lifestyle
  - Drawbacks of a permanent stoma and bag.
- Discuss the patient's fears:
  - Surgery
  - Permanent colostomy
  - Psychological implications.
- Discuss the available help – e.g. stoma nurse, self-help groups.

Directions of the consultation

Scenario A

He accepts what has been said.

- He should be allowed time to make a decision after consultation with other members of his family, if requested.
- Arrange a follow-up appointment or telephone discussion over the next day or so.

Scenario B

He is unwilling to have the procedure.

- Ultimately, it is the patient's decision, and under these circumstances he will continue to receive the best medical management without colostomy.
- Ask him if he would like to talk to someone else about the decision.
- Perhaps reach some form of compromise: 'We will give steroids one more go, and then reconsider matters.'
- Ensure he understands the implications of his decision and that colostomy is still an option for the future.
- Offer him time to discuss the issue further with family and friends. Candidates should not force a decision – you are not selling a time-share in Torremolinos.

Finishing

- Ask if he has understood everything that has been said and if he has any questions.
- Contact the multidisciplinary team for his next appointment.
- Make an appointment with the stoma nurse and/or other patients who have had a colectomy.

3.

You are the SHO in the renal clinic. A 54-year-old man has had type 2 diabetes for the last 15 years, which is poorly controlled. He also has hypertension and has been on continuous ambulatory peritoneal dialysis (CAPD) for the last 2 years. Previous haemodialysis has failed. He is not coping with CAPD.

Discuss with him the possibility of a renal transplant.

Preliminary thoughts

- Why is he not coping (e.g. false expectations, social, compliance, recurrent infections)?
- Advantages and disadvantages of CAPD vs. renal transplant
- Short-, medium- and long-term complications of renal transplant
- Practicalities of obtaining a transplant
- Legal and ethical issues:
  - Do patients with diabetes benefit from transplantation? Is it a good use of a limited resource? The answer to both is 'Yes'
  - It is illegal to buy and sell kidneys for transplantation in the UK
  - Should transplanted kidneys be allocated on a waiting list or where doctors perceive the greatest utility?

Goals of the consultation

- He must understand the benefits of changing from CAPD.
- He must understand the implications of transplantation.
- By the end of the consultation he should be in a position to make an informed decision about his future management.

Key points in the consultation

- Introduce yourself to the patient and establish rapport.
- Explore the patient's understanding of his condition.
- Discuss the reasons for non-coping with CAPD.
- Explore the patient's expectations of CAPD and transplantation.
- Explain that he has endstage renal failure and requires support. If he is not managing CAPD, renal transplantation is the only alternative, as haemodialysis has previously failed.

- Explain the practicalities of obtaining a transplant:
  - Cadaveric vs. live donor
  - The waiting list is long – cannot guarantee he will get one
  - The length of wait for transplant depends on finding an acceptable HLA match
  - Explain the complications of transplant:
  - Short-term complications – surgical risks
  - Medium-term complications:
    - immunosuppression – infection
    - risk of rejection
  - Long-term complications:
    - immunosuppression – secondary malignancy and infection
    - recurrent renal failure – 5-year graft survival (see *Transplantation*, p. 39).

Finishing

- Ensure the patient understands what has been said.
- Ask if he has any questions.
- Arrange a follow-up appointment.

4.

A 48-year-old man who is a company director has recently undergone a routine employment medical which has revealed glycosuria (no ketones). A subsequent fasting glucose level is 12 mmol/litre. He smokes 20 cigarettes/day, has a sedentary lifestyle and is obese. He has been referred to a new-patient diabetic clinic for further advice and management.

Please discuss this with him.

Preliminary thoughts

- Symptoms of hyperglycaemia
- Lifestyle influences
- Lifelong management
- Complications of diabetes
- Treatment options
- UKPDS (UK Prospective Diabetes Study) data

Goals of the consultation

- For him to understand the importance of the patient and doctor (as part of the multidisciplinary team) working together to control the disease (his input is vital).
- Ensure he understands the lifelong nature of the disease, its complications and the need for treatment and lifestyle modification to prevent these complications.

Key points in the consultation

- Introduce yourself to the patient and establish rapport.
- Establish the patient's understanding of diabetes and its implications.
- Establish the patient's expectations.
- Explain to the patient the basic mechanisms underlying his diabetes.
- Explain the aims of treatment – to reduce the risk of complications:
  - Macrovascular:
    - IHD, cerebrovascular and peripheral vascular disease
  - Microvascular:
    - nephropathy
    - retinopathy
    - neuropathy.

- All of these can be reduced with optimal glycaemic control.
- Explain the UKPDS data.
- Emphasise need for lifelong treatment.
- Emphasise the multidisciplinary approach:
  - Diabetic specialist nurse
  - Dietician
  - Chiropodist
  - Ophthalmologist
  - Need for teamwork, but the 'patient is the driver of the train'.
- Outline possible treatments:
  - Emphasising that dietary modification is the most important aspect of treatment, combined with exercise
  - Discuss oral medication if this is unsuccessful
  - Discuss the possibility of insulin therapy in the future.
- Address other risk factors, i.e. hypertension, hyperlipidaemia, smoking.
- Emphasise the need for compliance and regular review.

Finishing

- Introduce him to the diabetic team.
- Give him information about diabetes.
- Arrange patient education sessions.
- Arrange follow-up with the multidisciplinary team.

5.

A 55-year-old lady has recently entered the menopause. She has very troublesome hot flushes and some vaginal dryness. She has read about hormone replacement therapy (HRT) and wishes to discuss this with you. Her younger sister died 2 years ago of breast carcinoma.

Please discuss HRT with her.

Preliminary thoughts

- Pros and cons of HRT
- Risk vs. benefit – cancer, osteoporosis, symptoms, cardiovascular status
- Alternatives to HRT for symptoms
- Mammographic screening for breast cancer and its reduced efficacy with HRT
- Legal and ethical issues regarding informed consent

Goals of the consultation

- She must be in a position to make an informed decision.
- She must be aware of the increased risks in her particular case.
- Discuss alternative treatments (e.g. clonidine for hot flushes).

Key points in the consultation

- Introduce yourself to the patient and establish rapport.
- Establish the patient's knowledge of HRT and her concerns about it.
- Establish the patient's expectations.
- Explain the risks/benefits of HRT:
  - Benefits:
    - relieves symptoms of oestrogen deficiency
    - prevents osteoporosis
    - possible decrease in the risk of ischaemic heart disease, but evidence is unclear
    - decreases the risk of uterine carcinoma and possibly colonic carcinoma
  - Contraindications revolve predominantly around an increased risk of breast carcinoma. This is increased due to a family history. Oestrogens increase the risk of breast cancer approximately twofold, but sixfold with a family history.

- Discuss alternatives to HRT, e.g. clonidine for hot flushes, evening primrose oil, topical oestrogens.
- Explain the need for annual mammograms and self-examination.
- Explain that HRT will result in her continuing to have regular withdrawal bleeds that she may find troublesome.
- Ultimately, the decision is the patient's and she needs to weigh up the theoretical risks and inconvenience against her troublesome symptoms.

Directions of the consultation

Scenario A

She has made her mind up and ultimately wants treatment.

- Under these circumstances the patient should be aware of the possible risks, and these should be carefully documented in her notes.
- Due to the great increase in the potential risk of cancer, it is advisable to arrange another consultation to discuss this further.
- If the doctor feels that he is ethically unable to prescribe the drug then she should seek a second opinion.

Scenario B

She remains unsure what to do and is looking for advice.

- Under these circumstances she should be made aware of the increased risks and encouraged initially to try alternatives, with a regular follow-up arrangement.

Finishing

- Ensure she understands all the issues.
- Ask if she has any questions.
- Everything should be carefully documented in the notes.
- If she has decided to try HRT, she must be aware of the gravity of her decision.
- Follow-up arrangements should be made in both cases.

6.

An 84-year-old man has been admitted to hospital, having been found collapsed and confused at home. He lives alone in a warden-controlled flat. On admission 2 weeks ago he had a mental test score (MTS) of 1/10, but after treatment of his urinary tract infection he now has a MTS of 8/10. The medical and nursing staff think he is safe to go home and he has been assessed by the occupational therapist and physiotherapist with a successful home visit. The patient wishes to return home, but his daughter is extremely concerned about him and refuses to let him home. The daughter has made an appointment to see you to discuss her father.

Please discuss the situation with her.

Preliminary thoughts

- Avoid antagonising the daughter; keep her onside.
- Keep control in a non-confrontational manner.
- What are her concerns/worries?
- Need for flexibility and compromise with the daughter.
- Legal and ethical issues – the daughter has no legal rights over the care of her father, although she may be heavily involved at home. It is important to respect her opinion, but ultimately the decision must be made in the best interests of the patient, not the daughter.

Goals of the consultation

- To follow the patient's wishes and enable him to go home.
- Explore why the daughter doesn't agree.
- To make her aware of the reasons as to why he should go home.
- To ultimately gain her support on his returning home.

Key points in the consultation

- Introduce yourself to the patient and establish rapport.
- Explore her knowledge and views of her father's medical and social circumstances and why she feels he is unsafe to return home.
- Explore her real reasons – social needs, guilt. For example, she may not be able to look after him at home for that particular week only; under these circumstances a compromise can be sought.

- Explain his medical condition and that it is now fully treated, that his condition has now returned to his pre-admission state but is unlikely to improve further.
- Explain that he has been assessed by the multidisciplinary team (occupational therapy, physiotherapy and social worker), all of whom think he is safe to go home.
- Explain the risks of staying in hospital (e.g. chest infections, immobility).
- Determine what can be done to get her to change her mind.
- Explain that your duty of care is to the patient, who wants to go home.
- He may be eligible for additional help:
  - Home help
  - Meals-on-wheels
  - Attendance at a day centre
  - Explain that he will be carefully observed with a follow-up appointment.

Directions of the consultation

Scenario A

She remains adamant that he should stay in hospital.

- Under these circumstances a form of compromise or trial period at home can be attempted.
- The daughter must be made aware that it is in the patient's best interests to go home, but if things do not work out the situation can be reassessed.
- Impress on her that he will have continuing care and follow-up in the community and that hospitals are not necessarily the safest place to be.
- Arrange a case conference of all involved parties.

Scenario B

There is something specific troubling her.

- The doctor should address this point and attempt to solve it.

Finishing

- Ask if she has any further questions.
- Agree a date for him returning home.
- Arrange for further discussions, if requested.
- Ensure the nurses and team in the community are aware of the situation and your discussions.

7.

A 22-year-old man has recently noticed a lump in his left testicle. Ultrasound was highly suspicious of malignancy, which was confirmed histologically (germ-cell tumour) after unilateral orchidectomy. CT staging has shown local lymph node involvement, which will require cytotoxic chemotherapy; with the correct treatment his chance of long-term survival is greater than 90%.

Please discuss with the patient his diagnosis and need for chemotherapy.

Preliminary thoughts

- Underlying diagnosis is cancer
- What does he know or suspect?
- Good prognosis
- Treatment
- Fertility issues – reduced with chemotherapy

Goals of the consultation

- Establish his current understanding of his condition.
- Explain his diagnosis to him.
- Ensure he understands the need for chemotherapy and the good prognosis.
- Ensure follow-up and support.

Key points in the consultation

- Introduce yourself to the patient and establish rapport.
- Ask if he wants anyone else present.
- Establish the patient's views on what he thinks might be the diagnosis and what he knows.
- Determine which category he falls into (whether he wants all the information at once or is a 'nugget' type – see *Breaking bad news*, p. 273).
- Once the patient's understanding of the condition has been established, it is possible to predict if he is expecting a diagnosis of cancer.

Directions of the consultation

Scenario A

He is aware that testicular cancer is a possibility.

- The patient should be informed of the diagnosis in a clear and sympathetic manner. He may wish to see his CT scans or the histology report, which is sometimes helpful.
- Explain the nature of the disease, the need for cyclical combination chemotherapy over a period of several weeks and its side-effects.
- Explain that treatment will give him a very good outcome.

Scenario B

The patient has not considered cancer as a possible diagnosis.

- The patient should be given small pieces of information at a time, working towards the diagnosis.
- The doctor should be relatively positive, as the outcome is usually good with chemotherapy.
- Remember that once the patient has been told his diagnosis, he should be allowed time to react.
- Pause before moving on.
- Explain the need for subsequent cytotoxic chemotherapy:
  - Logistics – when, where, frequency (he should start very soon)
  - Side-effects, e.g. infection, alopecia, nausea, infertility.
- Discuss the sequelae of his condition:
- Cosmetic – testicular prosthesis can be inserted.
- Fertility – unaffected by previous surgery, likely to be infertile after chemotherapy, but semen can be frozen and stored.
- Need for future monitoring of response to treatment:
  - CT body
  - Blood tests – HCG/AFP/LDH.
- Emphasise the very good prognosis for testicular cancer; >90% cure.

Finishing

- Ask the patient if he understands what has been said.
- Summarise the consultation.
- Ask if he has any questions.

- Arrange medical follow-up.
- Arrange a point of contact (e.g. telephone no.) with the oncology nurse specialist.
- Make sure there is someone he can talk to, or someone at home with him.

8.

You are the respiratory SHO. The next patient is a 39-year-old poorly controlled asthmatic who has been placed on long-term oral steroids by your consultant. The patient is very worried about the steroids as she has read that they make her weight increase and they do 'terrible things to your body'. The patient is also an insulin-dependent diabetic.

Please explain the steroid therapy to the patient.

Preliminary thoughts

- Benefits vs. side-effects of steroids (short- and long-term)
- Implications regarding diabetes
- Need for clear information
- Possible alternatives to steroids
- Legal and ethical issues – patients have the right to refuse treatment

Goals of the consultation

- She should understand the overwhelming benefit of steroids.
- She should accept the medical advice with a minimum of compromise, as this may lead to serious adverse consequences.

Key points in the consultation

- Polite introduction and establish rapport.
- Establish this patient's understanding of her disease and the need for steroids.
- Determine specifically why she does not want to take them and her anxieties about future use.
- Emphasise the need for steroids to prevent attacks and the consequences of poorly controlled asthma.
- Explain the possible long-term side-effects of steroids:
  - Weight gain
  - Thin skin
  - Bruising
  - Possible hypertension
  - Acne
  - Osteoporosis

- That these will be minimised by ensuring her dose is tailored to her condition. Osteoporosis can be minimised by concomitant bisphosphonate therapy.
- Explain the following about the therapy:
  - It will result in adrenal suppression and the absence of endogenous cortisol production
  - She should never stop the tablets suddenly
  - She must never miss a dose
  - If unwell she should double the dose for 72 hours. If she remains unwell she needs to seek medical attention
  - Need for a steroid card, medic alert bracelet and an emergency hydrocortisone pack (for parenteral self-administration if she's unable to take oral medication).
- Explain the effects on her diabetes and possible worsening of glycaemic control. She will probably need to increase her insulin dose, in liaison with her diabetologist/diabetic specialist nurse.

Finishing

- Ensure the patient understands what has been said and ask if she has any questions.
- Summarise what has been discussed.
- Arrange follow-up.

Discussion

The key to this is compliance with medication. A one-sided teacher/ student discussion is unlikely to result in good compliance. The doctor and patient should work together as a team. Ultimately, a discussion about reducing the dose to ensure compliance may be appropriate.

9.

As a cardiology SHO you know there is a long waiting list of patients for coronary intervention. Your next patient is a 52-year-old man who, despite having had two previous myocardial infarctions and a coronary artery bypass graft (CABG) 5 years ago, continues to smoke 40 cigarettes per day. He is now having recurrent worsening angina, with an exercise tolerance of 50 m. An angiogram shows diffuse disease not amenable to angio-plasty, but suitable for re-do CABG.

Please discuss the results of this test and further management. He is on maximal medical therapy.

Preliminary thoughts

- A re-do CABG may alleviate symptoms, but the risk vs. benefit must be considered
- Effects on his overall prognosis
- Does his lifestyle affect the decision vis-...-vis smoking?
- Attitude of patient and compliance with treatment
- Any previous attempts to stop smoking (nicotine gum, acupuncture, peer pressure)

Goals of the consultation

- He must understand that life modification is required (i.e. stopping smoking), as this itself will adversely affect his outcome.
- He must understand the morbidity and mortality associated with or without surgery.
- He must be aware that further intervention may not happen immediately (the waiting list principle associated with limited resources).

Key points in the consultation

- Introduce yourself and establish rapport.
- Establish this patient's understanding of his disease, its severity and consequences of continuing to smoke.
- Avoid being judgemental about his smoking.
- Explain the results of his recent angiogram.
- Establish this patient's understanding and expectations of his possible treatment options.

- Explain the risks and benefit of repeat CABG:
  - Possible relief of symptoms
  - Limited benefit in 5-year survival.
- Explore other treatment options, e.g. transcutaneous electrical nerve stimulation (TENS).
- Ensure other risk factors have been addressed.

Directions of the consultation

The doctor can approach the consultation in one of many ways, which will be influenced by both his own views and the attitude of the patient. The doctor should try and avoid preaching or being judgemental. The patient should be made aware that there is a need to stop smoking. However, there are ethical issues regarding whether his future management should depend on him agreeing to give up.

There are two extremes and most doctors' approach tends to be somewhere in the middle.

Scenario A

We will not go ahead with the surgery unless you agree to stop smoking. Reason: The money could probably be better spent on individuals who have stopped or never smoked.

Scenario B

You probably should try to give up, but we will put you on the waiting list anyway.
Reason: He has paid his National Insurance contributions (and a large amount of tax on cigarettes) and therefore deserves the same care as everyone else. After all, there is no guarantee that once the procedure has taken place the patient will not start smoking again, even if he promises to give up.

Finishing

- Ensure he understands the need to stop smoking and the possibility of further surgery.
- Summarise the consultation.
- Ask if he has any questions.
- Arrange follow-up.

10.

A 48-year-old taxi driver who has type 2 diabetes is attending your diabetic clinic. He has had multiple laser photocoagulations for pre-proliferative retinopathy and now has a fixed-field defect that does not fulfil DVLA requirements for driving. He says that he cannot afford to give up driving as he is the only income earner in the family and has three small children.

Please discuss this with him.

Preliminary thoughts

- His legal obligation to inform the DVLA
- The ethical reasons why he should stop driving – danger to others
- Your ethical and legal obligations as a doctor
- Social implications – alternative careers
- His right to ask for a second opinion

Goals of the consultation

- Impress upon him the need to stop driving (legal and ethical issues).
- Maintain the doctor–patient relationship, so he will return to the clinic.
- He informs the DVLA.

Key points in the consultation

- Introduce yourself to the patient and establish rapport.
- Establish the patient's expectations and understanding of diabetes and driving.
- Explain the results of his visual field tests and their implications.
- Approach the consultation in a manner of the doctor and patient working together as a team.
- Establish why the patient 'cannot afford' to stop driving.
- Look for a possible compromise, e.g. enlist social services help for alternative careers and financial support.
- Impress on him the danger to himself and others if he continues to drive.
- If necessary, raise issues of family and social obligation.
- Inform the patient of his legal obligation to inform the DVLA; if he will not, you will have to.

Finishing

- Write careful records of all the discussions in the notes.
- Summarise the consultation.
- Ensure he understands what has been said.
- Ask if he has any questions.
- Arrange a follow-up appointment.

Discussion

In this scenario, the worse case is if the patient leaves the consultation and continues to drive illegally and does not return. You need to strike a balance between firmness and empathy. This scenario again emphasises the need for candidates in PACES to be familiar with both the law regarding driving, and the common medical conditions that legally prevent driving (*www.dvla.gov.uk*), see p. 115 and 295. The same DVLA rules apply to taxi drivers as to other motor vehicle users, although they are additionally subject to restrictions from the Public Carriage Office/ Local Authority.

11.

As a medical SHO, you are looking after a 74-year-old man who was admitted with a GI bleed. Subsequent endoscopy has shown this was due to an underlying gastric carcinoma and a CT scan has demonstrated widespread metastatic disease. He is a widower who has repeatedly stated that he does not want any intervention. The psychiatrist has reviewed him and has stated that he is not depressed. He has now had a further GI bleed and is alert but clinically shocked. He is still refusing further intervention.

Please discuss this further with him.

Preliminary thoughts

- Does the patient understand the gravity of the situation?
- Legal position of the patient – informed consent and the right to refuse treatment – e.g. blood transfusion.
- Legal position of the doctor – treating a patient against their will is battery.
- Treatment options available – palliative (no treatment should be given to accelerate death. However, treatment for symptoms, with side-effects, can be given, e.g. morphine).
- Is there anyone else he would like contacted?

Goals of the consultation

- Patient understands the seriousness of his condition.
- The patient makes a truly informed decision.
- Ensure other members of the medical and nursing team are aware of his decision.

Key points in the consultation

- Introduce yourself to the patient and establish a good rapport.
- Explore the patient's feelings as to why he refuses treatment.
- Explore the patient's understanding of his underlying diagnosis and prognosis.
- Explore the patient's understanding of what refusal will entail, i.e. probable death within hours.

- Explain the possible treatment options:
    - Immediate for the bleeding – transfusion, sclerotherapy or laser photocoagulation; surgery is not a viable option
    - Pain control, anxiolytics.
- Inform the patient that you will comply with his wishes, even if he becomes unconscious.
- Ask the patient if he has told other members of the family, or if he would like them to know of his decision.
- Ask if he has sorted out his affairs at home as things may get suddenly worse.
- Ask if there is anyone he would like to be informed or contacted.
- Inform nursing and on-call teams.

Finishing

- Carefully document the discussion in the notes.
- Summarise what has been discussed.
- Ask if he has any questions.
- Ensure all has been done to improve his symptoms.

Discussion

This scenario tests your understanding of informed consent, and you need to consider how an advance directive would affect the situation (see p. 283). You are not being tested on the emergency treatment of a shocked patient.

12.

As a medical registrar, you have been looking after an 18-year-old boy on ITU since he was knocked off his bicycle 1 week ago. He has been on a life-support machine since admission. You have agreed with the father (the sole carer) the need to do brainstem tests and he has made an appointment with you to discuss the results. The tests have confirmed that his son is brainstem dead.

Please inform the father of the results and discuss organ donation with him. The son did not carry a donor card.

Preliminary thoughts

- What are brainstem tests? (see p. 286)
- Legalities of declaring someone dead
- What organ donation entails and the need for consent from the next of kin/relative (see p. 289).
- Which organs? – speed, need, number of patients who will benefit
- Rules surrounding donor cards/advance directives
- Will the father need other family members present to help make a decision?

Goals of the consultation

- The father understands his son is dead.
- An informed decision has to be made relatively soon about organ donation.

Key points in the consultation

- Introduce yourself and establish a good rapport.
- Ask if he would like anyone else there for the discussion.
- Explore and confirm the father's understanding of his son's condition.
- Confirm his acceptance of his son's dependency on life-support machines and why the tests were done.

The subsequent direction of the consultation depends on the father's acceptance of the previous point.

Directions of the consultation

Scenario A

The father is unaware or does not accept that his son might be dead.

- This is a difficult situation; the doctor should go through the information piece by piece, starting from the beginning when he arrived in ITU. The doctor should pause frequently to allow the father time to think and ask any questions. Ultimately, it is essential that the father knows his son is dead. He may need more time to take this in and it may be inappropriate to discuss organ donation at this stage.
- The father should therefore be given some time to discuss the situation with family and friends, and then a subsequent discussion regarding organ transplantation would be appropriate.

Scenario B

The father is aware of the reasons why the tests are being performed and their significance.

- Inform him of the test results, i.e. brainstem death. Confirm there is no hope of recovery; the son is being kept in his current state by the ventilator.
- Explore the father's knowledge of organ donation.
- Did the son ever discuss his feelings regarding organ donation?
- Offer details regarding organ donation and the benefits to a number of other individuals. The shortage of hearts, lungs, kidneys, for example, which may enable other people to live who would otherwise die.
- Remember this is not an all-or-nothing situation – relatives, who are legal guardians of the body, may specify which are acceptable or unacceptable organs for donation.
- Offer him the opportunity to have a further discussion with other members of the family; arrange to meet again in the next few hours.

Finishing

- Ask the father if there is anyone else he would like to inform.
- Ask if he has any questions.
- Ensure all staff involved in the case are aware of the father's decision.

Discussion

- The examiners may wish to discuss the difference between brainstem death and persistent vegetative state (see p. 287).
- Discussions with relatives are often best done in a group to ensure a consensus is reached. Focusing on one relative may lead to jealousy and resentment. However, if it becomes apparent that differing views are held by different members, you may need to deal with a 'spokesperson' who will act for all family members.

13.

An 80-year old man, previously alert and independent, has been brought in with a massive haemoptysis. He has been resuscitated and bronchoscopy has revealed a probable bronchial carcinoma, but histology is awaited. Ultrasound shows multiple liver metastases, but an enhanced CT head scan is normal. He remains acutely confused, but his wife is understandably anxious and wishes to know what is going on. She has, as yet, been told very little information.

Please discuss her husband's condition with her.

Preliminary thoughts

- Legal vs. pragmatic issues regarding patient confidentiality and when it can be broken (see p. 283)
- Prognosis:
  - Short-term – moderate
  - Medium-term – very poor
- Need to reassure wife regarding her husband's care
- Prepare her for bad news

Goals of the consultation

- The wife must be made aware that he is very unwell, although exact details of his condition may be unnecessary.
- To ensure the wife has faith in the medical care her husband is receiving.

Key points in the consultation

- Introduce yourself and establish a good rapport.
- 'Ideally, we would have this discussion with your husband too, but it is not possible. You must be very anxious.'
- What has she been told already?
- Establish the wife's knowledge of her husband's condition and why she thinks he is in hospital.
- Inform her that he has had a large haemoptysis, but that this has been treated and he should recover from his confusion.

The subsequent direction of the consultation depends on the under-standing and expectations of the wife. The doctor should now pause to let the wife ask questions.

Directions of the consultation

Scenario A

The wife has no comprehension of how serious the condition may be.

- Under these circumstances the wife should be informed that her husband is unwell. It should be impressed on her that the situation is serious and that further discussion with her and ideally her husband will be required in the near future.
- Allow her to ask any questions. Answer these as honestly as possible. It should be remembered that the histology is still awaited and a diagnosis of cancer, although likely, has not been confirmed.
- Discussing the diagnosis of cancer without histology is hazardous and best avoided.
- It is never appropriate to force information on patients or relatives.
- Although discussing her husband's details is technically breaking patient confidentiality, most clinicians would agree that discussing with the wife is the correct ethical thing to do. The amount of detail will, of course, depend on her questions and reaction to the answers.
- Legally, this is permissible since the clinician is acting in the best interests of the patient as she may be aware of his wishes in such situations.
- Moreover, it would be generally accepted that it is also humane to let his partner know of his condition.

Scenario B

It is clear from talking to the wife that she is aware something is seriously amiss; the thought of cancer may have crossed her mind.

- Remember the diagnosis has not been confirmed and that the patient's confusion is likely to improve. Predicting the future is difficult and best avoided.
- Doctors should attempt to maintain a degree of confidentiality in telling the wife what she wants to know (e.g. 'One of the tests show there is something suspicious in his lungs; it may be a serious problem, although we are not absolutely sure of that yet.').

- In view of the lack of definite histology, the authors feel that discussing resuscitation with the wife at this stage is inappropriate and the patient should remain for resuscitation. However, if the wife volunteers that her husband would not like further intervention if something went suddenly wrong, this should be considered, together with the subsequent results of the histology.

Finishing

- Summarise the consultation.
- Ask if she has any questions.
- Arrange a further meeting.
- Inform the nursing staff of the conversation – they should ideally have been present.

Discussion

As with many communication skills' scenarios, particularly those relating to imparting bad news, the wife dictates the direction, pace and flow of the consultation.

14.

A 33-year-old lady has a consultation with you to discuss the results of her recent MRI scan, which you had organised at her previous neurology appointment. She has a 3-year-old daughter and is actively trying for a second child. For the last 3 months she has noticed several episodes of visual disturbance and intermittent weakness of her legs. Her MRI scan is consistent with the diagnosis of multiple sclerosis.

Please discuss this result with her.

Preliminary thoughts

- The course of MS and its variable nature
- Morbidity and mortality of MS
- Implications regarding pregnancy
- Treatment options, including beta-interferon and the NICE guidelines
- Inheritance of MS

Goals of the consultation

For her to understand:
- The diagnosis and its implications
- The need for a multidisciplinary approach
- The variable nature of progression of the disease; few patients progress rapidly
- Treatment options.

Key points in the consultation

- Introduce yourself to the patient and establish good rapport.
- Ask if she wishes for anyone else to be present.
- Explore the patient's understanding of her condition and expectations/suspicions of what may be wrong.

Directions of the consultation

Scenario A

The patient has never heard of MS and has no idea of its implications.

- The patient should be given small pieces of information in a logical manner; pauses are essential and give the opportunity for questions.

- Patients can be given too much information in one consultation after receiving bad news. It is preferable to establish one or two key points.
- Further consultations can address more detailed information. They may choose to bring a friend or relative.

Scenario B

The patient is suspicious that MS is the cause and knows a great deal about it.

A discussion about exactly what she understands and expects is important. The press tend to report the more disabling end of the disease spectrum, heightening patient anxiety.
- Emphasise the variable progression of the disease. Often remitting/relapsing. There can be long periods with few symptoms. Few patients progress rapidly.
- Discuss available treatment options such as steroids and beta-interferon (in outline only), see p. 142.
- Discuss the implications for pregnancy and whether this should be pursued – MS has no effect on fertility and does not affect pregnancy outcome.
- Reassure her that it is not hereditary.

Finishing

- Summarise what has been discussed.
- Ask if there is anything she would like repeated or if she has any questions.
- Arrange follow-up and put her in touch with support groups.

Discussion

- Patients do not absorb masses of information from consultations. This is worse in anxious situations. For this reason it is preferable to give and repeat a little information well, to write it down if possible and to arrange to discuss issues further at the next appointment. Having a relative or friend present is reassuring and helps in the amount of information recalled.
- It is always best to give a little information well than a lot badly.

15.

You have admitted a 74-year-old man to a general medical ward with a chest infection. He has known pre-existing ischaemic heart failure (NYHA grade 3), for which he is receiving optimum medical therapy. The staff nurse has bleeped you to clarify his resuscitation status, as there is no written record.

Please discuss this issue with your patient.

Preliminary thoughts

- Resuscitation (see p. 288)
- Risk vs. benefit
- His irreversible medical condition with limited life expectancy
- Low likelihood of success
- Legal and ethical issues – the best practice is that patients' resuscitation status should be discussed with them whenever possible (a view endorsed by the GMC). A possible exception to this is when resuscitation is deemed futile

Goals of the consultation

- The patient makes an informed decision.
- Other member of the medical and nursing team are informed of this decision.

Key points in the consultation

- Introduce yourself to the patient and establish rapport.
- Ensure you are in a correct setting – patient on his own, with staff nurse present.
- Establish the patient's understanding of his underlying condition and reason for admission.
- Emphasise that he is on maximum medical therapy which will continue.
- What does he think will happen in the future?
- He should be aware that there will be a relentless decline in his cardiac function.

At this point pause and allow the patient to reflect on the discussion.

Directions of the consultation

Scenario A

The patient is unaware of the seriousness of his underlying condition and still hopes for an improvement.

- Although this may be unrealistic, the patient's views should be respected.
- Gently ensure he is told of the seriousness of his condition.
- If he feels strongly that he would like every medical attempt made to prolong his life, then that should also be respected.
- The issue of resuscitation should be addressed directly, once the patient understands his serious and progressive condition:
  - 'We should address what you would like us to do if your health was to take a sudden turn for the worse?'
- Hopefully by this stage, the doctor and patient will have established a rapport that does not make the question seem out of place.

Scenario B

The patient understands the seriousness of condition, but is unsure whether resuscitation would be appropriate.

- Often the patient will ask: 'What do you think doctor?'
- The patient should be informed of the relatively poor outcome of resuscitation and the often undignified manner of death (risks vs. benefits).

Scenario C

The patient has thought about his condition and does not want resuscitation.

- His view should be respected and documented in his notes.
- The patient should be asked if he has discussed it with his next of kin, although this is not legally necessary.

Scenario D

The patient may leave the decision in the hands of the doctor.

- If this is the case the medical and nursing team should make a decision together.
- The patient should be asked if they want their relatives involved or even told.

Finishing

- Summarise the consultation.
- Ask the patient if they have understood the discussion and if they have any questions.
- Inform the nursing staff.
- Document the decision carefully in the notes.

Discussion

- Decisions about the cardiopulmonary resuscitation (CPR) status of patients should be made whenever possible in full consultation with them.
- It should be borne in mind that for every patient there comes a time when death is inevitable and cardiac or respiratory function will fail. It is essential therefore to determine, for each patient, whether CPR is appropriate.
- Detailed up-to-date guidelines are provided by the Resuscitation Council of the UK (*www.resus.org.uk/pages/dnar*).
- The principles are that effective, sensitive communication with patients should be undertaken in advance, keeping in mind that the circumstance of every patient is unique. Information about CPR and the chances of a successful outcome should be realistic.
- A 'Do not attempt resuscitation' (DNAR) order should only be given after full consultation with the patient and the medical team.
- Situations in which it is not necessary to discuss with patients include those where attempting CPR will be unsuccessful, or where there would be no benefit, e.g. coexistent severe morbidity.

16.

As a general medical SHO you discover that one of your patients with pyelonephritis was given too much gentamicin over the weekend, despite documented levels being toxic. She has since developed ototoxicity and deteriorating renal function, but is unlikely to need dialysis.

Please discuss the situation with the patient.

Preliminary thoughts

- Above all, do not lie or cover up.
- Most patients understand human fallibility and that no one is perfect.
- Potentially, expect a stormy consultation.
- Determine the precise circumstances around the error before the consultation and discuss with the relevant people what happened.
- This is not about apportioning blame or pointing the finger.

Goals for consultation

- To have a frank and truthful discussion.
- For the patient to feel:
  - That the matter is being dealt with appropriately and adequately
  - Plans are being made to prevent it happening again.

Key points in the consultation

- Introduce yourself to the patient and establish rapport.
- Tell the patient that there has been a problem with one of the drugs she was given.
- Explain the concept of a therapeutic range for gentamicin and the need to monitor levels.
- Explain what happened and how.
- Apologise for the error.
- Emphasise openness and truthfulness.
- Explain the side-effects of gentamicin.
- Natural history – renal function will probably recover, but the ototoxicity may not.
- Explain the steps you have taken to determine the cause and to prevent it happening again.
- Inform her you will arrange for an ENT and a renal opinion.

- Explain the need for continuing medical care for the pyelonephritis.
- Explain the possibility of further action for her to take in the future, e.g. formal complaint.

Discussion

In circumstances of medical malpractice there are several key issues. The most important, above all, is to be apologetic and truthful. Do not:

- Lie
- Cover up
- Be evasive
- Alter notes
- Point the finger.

Although, it may be tempting to try and tell half-truths or cover up mistakes in a patient's management, the truth should be told. In any case, it almost inevitably comes out at some stage. Two erroneous ways in which to lead this scenario are either to try and pretend that an error was not made – 'We have got the levels of the gentamicin back now. They were a little bit high and that might have caused some of the problems,' or to point the finger at someone else – 'Someone is going down for this, and it is not going to be me.'

✓

17.

You are the SHO in the endocrine clinic. The biochemical results on the next patient, a 32-year-old woman, confirm the clinical suspicion that she has Graves' disease, with a grossly elevated free T_4 and suppressed TSH with strongly positive antithyroid antibodies. She has moderate exophthalmos and is a smoker.

Please discuss with her the subsequent management of her condition.

Preliminary thoughts

- Treatment options of thyrotoxicosis and the pros and cons of each:
  - Medical – carbimazole, propylthiouracil
  - Radioiodine
  - Surgical
- Involve her in discussion
- Fertility issues

Goals of the consultation

- Inform her about her disease and discuss the management options.
- Agree the appropriate treatment strategy.
- Ensure she understands the seriousness of her condition and the need for regular monitoring.

Key points in the consultation

- Introduce yourself and establish rapport.
- Explore her knowledge of thyrotoxicosis.
- Explain the results of the blood test.
- Explain the nature of an overactive thyroid and the pathological consequences of untreated disease.
- Discuss the treatment options.
- Explain that her symptoms will improve with treatment, but may take months to resolve completely.
- If medical therapy, warn of the potential side-effects, especially agranulocytosis. This must be given both verbally and in writing.
- Establish her last menstrual period (LMP), wishes for pregnancy and if she has any children. Emphasise the need for regular review.

Finishing

- Summarise what has been said.
- Provide written information.
- Ask if they have any questions.
- Arrange follow-up with blood tests.

Discussion

- There are three potential treatment possibilities for thyrotoxicosis, of varying appropriateness.
- The pros and cons of each modality should be discussed.
- However, initial discussions will be influenced by her thyrotoxic anxiety; informed consent is often difficult in a thyrotoxic patient (see p. 282).
- For an initial presentation of Graves' disease, most endocrinologists would recommend a course of medical therapy, e.g. carbimazole 40 mg once a day (initially) with additional β-blockade to cover/mask the sympathetic activity. Therapy for 18 months may lead to remission in 50% of patients. The dose of carbimazole should be titrated according to thyroid function tests. An alternative regime is to 'block and replace'. Definitive treatment may be necessary if there is recurrence.
- It is medicolegally essential to record that patients commenced on either carbimazole or propylthiouracil (PTU) have been warned of the side-effects, such as rash (1 in 200) and agranulocytosis (1 in 2,000), and to attend for a blood count if they experience a sore throat within the first 3 months on medication.
- Early radioiodine (I-131) is an alternative after the patient is rendered euthyroid.
- Radioiodine is obviously contraindicated in pregnancy, and conception should not occur within 6 months. Close contact with small children is forbidden for several days after ingestion.
- Surgery offers a definitive cure, but leaves a scar and the possibility of recurrent laryngeal nerve damage, as well as hypoparathyroidism (more common with total thyroidectomy).
- The latter two treatments may render the patient hypothyroid, so requiring hormone replacement for life.
- Thyroid disease and pregnancy is the realm of specialists. Thyrotoxicosis decreases the chance of conceiving and increases the risk of spontaneous miscarriage. In Graves' disease, the stimulating antibodies can cross the placenta causing fetal thyrotoxicosis. Alternatively, both carbimazole and PTU can cross the placenta, so causing fetal hypothyroidism and goitre formation.

18.

You are a medical SHO in the neurology clinic. The next patient is a 36-year-old woman who has had a genetic test for Huntington's chorea and who has returned today for the result. She had previously found out that her father committed suicide aged 50 when he was diagnosed as having the disorder, but none of her three brothers know about their father's condition. She has two daughters, aged 4 and 7 years. The test indicates that she has the disorder (she is heterozygous).

Please counsel the patient with a view to discussing screening the rest of her family.

Preliminary thoughts

- She should have been consented appropriately for the genetic test and thus should understand the nature of the disease and implications of the result. However, this must not be taken for granted, even if you gained her consent yourself.
- The median age of onset of disease symptoms is between 30 and 45 years. Life expectancy is only 10 years after the onset of the symptoms. Chorea tends to occur first, and dementia a few years later.
- Should she tell her siblings about her diagnosis? Are any of her brothers planning on starting a family; if so, the need to inform them is probably greater, although, ultimately, confidentiality should be respected.
- What are the implications for her children?
- Tell her of the support groups for Huntington's disease and give her patients' information about it.

Goals of the consultation

- She must be aware of her diagnosis.
- She must understand the nature of the disease and its inheritance pattern.
- She should be put in contact with the relevant support groups.

Key points in the consultation

- Introduce yourself to the patient and establish rapport.
- Ask if she would like someone with her.
- Establish the patient's understanding of Huntington's chorea and its inheritance.
- Explore why she has had the test now.
- At this point the patient must understand the nature of the disease she is being tested for. She must be aware of the seriousness of the condition and its untreatable nature. If she is not fully aware, the doctor should discuss the nature of the disease at length with her.
- Before moving on, ask if she has any questions about the disease.
- Explain that the test is positive.
- At this point await for the patient's reaction, which may range from passive acceptance to tearful anger, through to questioning as to its significance and what it means.

Directions of the consultation

Scenario A

She is not emotionally well prepared.

- The patient may display a wide range of emotions, including tears, anger or denial.
- Initially, it really is just a case of listening and answering questions.
- The patient may not wish to talk about siblings or children at this point, although she may already be aware of the inherited nature of the disease.
- As in other cases of breaking bad news, all the information should not necessarily be forced upon her at this consultation, if she is not prepared for it.

Scenario B

The patient is well prepared and may be very accepting and matter-of-fact about the diagnosis.

- She may have a list of questions she wants answering. Doctors should do their best to answer them truthfully.
- If appropriate and depending on the patient's response, she should be asked if she has thought about telling other members of her family, the implications of the inheritance and who may or may not

be affected (the patient may not wish to discuss this, but it should be addressed at follow-up visits).
- Discuss support groups.
- Ensure the patient has adequate emotional support at home.

Finishing

- Summarise the discussion.
- Ask if she has any further questions.
- Arrange follow-up.

Discussion

- The disease is autosomal dominant and exhibits anticipation, whereby it occurs earlier and with greater severity in successive generations.
- Antenatal diagnosis from amniocentesis can be offered as appropriate.
- Pre-implantation *in vitro* diagnosis is a possibility.

19.

As a medical SHO, the on-call team informs you that a 73-year-old man under your care died during the night. He was admitted 48 hours earlier with pneumonia and appeared to be stable. Unfortunately, he deteriorated suddenly overnight and had an asystolic arrest. Attempted resuscitation was unsuccessful. The cause of death remains uncertain, although progressive pneumonia or pulmonary embolus is suspected. The daughter has been in close contact with her father during his admission, but was uncontactable last night. She has arrived on the ward and has been given a cup of tea in a private room for relatives; she is unaware that her father has died.

Please explain to her what has happened and enquire about the possibility of a postmortem.

Preliminary thoughts

- Was she aware that her father might die in hospital?
- Active management was attempted but was unsuccessful.
- The cause of death is uncertain, thus a postmortem is desirable.
- If one is unsure of the cause of death a coroner's opinion should be sought. He may be happy to have a death certificate completed without a postmortem.
- If a death certificate can be completed she can refuse a postmortem.
- Need to discuss with the nursing staff the daughter's relationship with her father and her expectations. Also enquire about other relatives and family dynamics.
- Ask the nursing staff to attend a consultation.

Goals of the consultation

For the daughter to understand:
- Her father has died despite the best efforts of the medical and nursing staff
- The cause of death probably relates to a respiratory disease
- The exact cause remains uncertain, making a postmortem desirable.

Key points in the consultation

- Ensure you will not be disturbed; give your pager to a colleague.
- Introduce yourself to the patient and establish rapport.
- Ask her if she would like anyone else present at this point.
- You must break the news about her father's death early on. You must provide the necessary background for this grave news, thus:
  - Explain the seriousness of pneumonia
  - Explore the daughter's knowledge and expectation of her father's illness, e.g. a good starting point being: 'How was he when you last saw him?'

Directions of the consultation

Scenario A

She is under the impression that all is well and he is likely to make a full and complete recovery.

- It is important to stress that her father's condition, although stable, was serious and deteriorated suddenly overnight. Attempts were made to contact her. It is now worth waiting once again for her reaction.
- She should be informed of the events that took place. The word 'death' should be used.
- She should be informed that full and active treatment was attempted, but was ultimately unsuccessful.
- During the consultation talk slowly, with empathy and appropriate pauses.
- Ask her if she would like some time alone or to contact friends/relatives.

Scenario B

She is aware that her father's condition is serious and was worried that he may deteriorate.

- Under these circumstances she should be informed that attempts were made to contact her last night.
- He deteriorated suddenly, resuscitation was attempted; however, this was unsuccessful and he died last night.
- If his death was swift and painless convey this to the relatives. Knowing the father did not suffer may be some comfort.

- It may or may not be appropriate at this point to discuss the postmortem, depending on her state of shock.
- If she would like to go on and discuss the postmortem further:
  - Explain that the doctors looking after her father would like to know exactly what caused the sudden deterioration. This can be done by performing a postmortem examination
  - The relatives need a general understanding of the procedure. Specific details are neither helpful nor necessary.

Finishing

- Give her your condolences.
- Ask if she has any questions.
- Ask if she would like to contact someone.
- Make follow-up arrangements to speak to her or other members of the family again, if necessary.

20.

As the SHO in infectious disease you are asked to see a 27-year-old female prostitute who had unprotected sex with her boyfriend the night before. She has subsequently discovered he is HIV-positive and has now attended the walk-in GU clinic for an HIV test and advice.

Please discuss these issues with her.

Preliminary thoughts

- Has she had an HIV test before?
- How does she know this other person has HIV?
- It takes 3 months to test HIV-positive after exposure.
- Hepatitis B and C should also be considered.
- Has she had Hep. B vaccine in the past?
- Has she put herself at risk of HIV before – unprotected sex with clients or IV drugs?
- She should be tested for HIV and Hep. B today and again in 3 months.
- She may benefit from receiving 3 months of prophylactic antiretroviral therapy (HAART) – this depends on whether she knows or not that her partner is HIV-positive; as antiretroviral medication carries an appreciable morbidity and mortality this should be discussed with an HIV physician.
- Hep. C should be tested for now and in 10 days – alpha-interferon will help clear viral antigen in acute infection.
- Is she pregnant?

Goals of the consultation

- The patient should be aware that there is an interim period of 3 months between exposure and testing positive. She should not put others at risk during this period.
- Discuss other viruses – hepatitis B and C.
- She should be aware of safe-sex practices.
- For her to understand that she may require prophylaxis against HIV.

Key points in the consultation

- Introduce yourself and try to establish a good rapport.
- The patient must be aware that confidentiality will be respected. However, confidentiality can be broken if she is knowingly putting others at risk.
- Discover the patient's knowledge about HIV, how it is transmitted and its prognosis.
- Depending on your rapport, try to ascertain why she is a prostitute – this may be important in terms of her future, e.g. IV drugs and coercion.
- Determine her use of IV drugs.
- How does she know her boyfriend is HIV-positive – confirmatory evidence?
- Avoid being judgemental.

Directions of the consultation

Scenario A

She is not prepared to discuss her private life – she just wants the test.

- Do not attempt to force information from her.
- She should be aware of the risk factors for becoming infected with HIV, and attempt to modify her lifestyle accordingly.
- Transmission rates for heterosexual sex are thought to be low in the UK and she should be relatively reassured, although a risk still exists.
- She should be counselled regarding the implications of testing positive:
  - Lifelong infection
  - Without treatment, relatively short life expectancy due to immune suppression
  - Thus increased risk of a variety of infections and cancers
  - New drugs have revolutionised the treatment with a marked improvement in life expectancy
  - However, no cure
  - Explain that she will also be tested for other viruses that she might be at risk of – hepatitis B and C
  - Having an HIV test may have implications for future life assurance, employment, etc., but it will be up to her to disclose this
  - Emphasise that her medical records are strictly confidential
  - If the test is positive, she will have to declare this on any future applications, if asked, or they will be invalid.

- She should understand the rationale behind 3 months' prophylactic antiretroviral therapy and its side-effects (common – rash, diarrhoea, allergy; uncommon – lactic acidosis, hepatitis, pancreatitis).
- She should be aware that she may be putting others at risk of HIV if she continues to have sex, until the result of the test is known. This may be difficult as it is her source of income.
- In any event, she should be told to always practise safe sex.

Scenario B

She is happy to discuss her life.

- Discuss her understanding of HIV infection and its risk factors.
- The relatively small chance of picking up HIV infection through this episode may be a low priority compared to other issues (IV drugs, accommodation, violence or sexual abuse). If appropriate, offer involvement of the social services and a multidisciplinary approach.
- Consent for an HIV test (see above).

Finishing

- Summarise what has been said.
- Ask if she has any questions.
- Make follow-up arrangements.
- Contact social services if required.

Discussion

- Remember that this is a test of communication skills. It is more important to appear sympathetic and non-judgemental than to know great details about the best combination of antiretroviral therapy.
- Some patients get constitutional symptoms during seroconversion that may be worth discussing.

STATION 5

The Skin, Locomotor, Eye and Endocrine Examinations

The Skin Examination

First let us consider the examination of the skin as a whole. Examine in good light, ideally natural light, and expose the patient as much as the situation will allow. Inspect the patient as a whole: look for any rash and consider its distribution, hair growth or loss and any features of systemic disease:

- Is there is a rash; is it red or not?
- Are there scales or evidence of excoriation?
- Is it macular, papular, in patches or plaques?
- Are there fluid-filled lesions, and are these vesicles, pustules or blisters?
- If you are pointed to a particular area examine this first, but be aware you may need to examine the skin as a whole as given below. (Where a specific condition is important it is mentioned.)
- Are there signs of systemic disease giving clues to the aetiology of the skin lesion, e.g. a colostomy bag?

One can see from the preceding list that there are numerous 'dermatological diagnoses' and numerous dermatological manifestations of systemic disease. The list is not exhaustive – consider for yourself what you might see as you examine a patient's skin and the associations of these cutaneous signs.

NAILS AND HANDS

- Pitting – psoriasis or fungal infection
- Onycholysis – psoriasis or thyrotoxicosis
- Paronychia – e.g. Cushing's disease or diabetes mellitus
- Pigmentation under the nail – possible subungual melanoma
- Splinter haemorrhages – vasculitis
- Telangiectasias – SLE
- Gottren's papules – purplish discoloration seen over the knuckles in dermatomyositis
- Blisters – seen in pemphigus and pemphigoid:
  - In pemphigus, fragile and may be open; in pemphigoid, tense
  - If the blisters are only on the hands consider photosensitivity, e.g. porphyria cutanea tarda
- Papules, scratch marks and tracks between the knuckles – scabies
- Viral warts – on the fingers or hands are common

- Dupuytren's contracture – alcoholics, familial and in operators of vibrating machinery
- Xanthomas – palmar creases and/or tendons
- Pigmentation – Addison's disease, particularly in the skin creases and knuckles; haemochromatosis; amiodarone therapy (slate-grey skin)
- Thin skin – Cushing's disease, with bruises and/or purpura

FOREARMS AND ARMS

- Lichen planus – on flexor surfaces, small, shiny purplish papules, Koebner phenomenon (scarring in scratch marks) may be seen as it is itchy
- Psoriasis – usually on extensor surfaces in silvery plaques
- Eczema – flexural with prominent excoriations
- Acanthosis nigricans – raised, dark, velvety areas of skin frequently in the axillas and neck, occurring in insulin resistance in polycystic ovary syndrome (PCOS), diabetes and also in solid malignancy
- Eruptive xanthomas – hypertriglyceridaemia (possible scars from operative management of acute pancreatitis)
- Dermatitis herpetiformis – blistering, extensor, itchy rash on extensor surfaces

HAIR AND SCALP

- Distribution of scalp hair:
  - Alopecia:
    - with normal skin, e.g. traction alopecia in nervous children, ringworm of the scalp (tinea capitis) or autoimmune alopecia areata (patchy hair loss)
    - scarring alopecia, e.g. discoid lupus, trigeminal zoster, burns
    - diffuse, temporary, hair loss is seen in patients treated with chemotherapy
  - Male-pattern hair loss with growth of body hair in women may point to virilising conditions, e.g. congenital adrenal hyperplasia
- Exclamation mark hairs – short hairs at the temples seen in SLE
- Dry, brittle hair – hypothyroidism
- Scaling – psoriasis, and in the navel
- Sebaceous cysts in the scalp are common

EYEBROWS AND EYELIDS

- Greasy and scaling – seborrhoeic dermatitis
- Heliotrope rash – seen in dermatomyositis on the eyelids and easily missed
- Xanthelasma – in types IIa and IIb hyperlipidaemia

FACE

- Capillary haemangiomas – Sturge–Weber syndrome, in a division of the trigeminal nerve, usually ophthalmic; may be associated with intracerebral AVM
- Rosacea – bright erythema on the nose, cheeks, forehead and chin
- Rhinophyma – disfiguring swelling of the nose
- Acne vulgaris – papules, pustules and scarring on the face, neck and upper trunk
- Butterfly rash – SLE; look closely for fine scales which plug the follicles as this is diagnostic
- Lupus pernio – dark-red discoloration of the nose in sarcoidosis
- Ulceration:
  - Basal-cell carcinoma
  - Squamous-cell carcinoma
  - Lupus vulgaris – tuberculosis (looks like apple jelly if a glass slide is pressed against the lesion)
- Keratoacanthoma– benign; volcano-like lesion arising out of a sebaceous gland
- Vesicles in a division of the trigeminal nerve – herpes zoster
- Lipodystrophy – with antiretroviral therapy in HIV-positive patients

LIPS/MOUTH

- Osler–Weber–Rendu (hereditary haemorrhagic telangiectasia)
- Peutz–Jeghers' syndrome
- Addison's disease – diffuse pigmentation next to the teeth (postural hypotension)
- Fissured lips with ulceration – Crohn's disease
- Herpes simplex

NECK/TRUNK

- Loose folds of redundant chicken skin – pseudoxanthoma elasticum
- Lymphadenopathy – where is it draining – infection or primary malignancy? Look closely at the scalp/face (and in the mouth)
- Depigmentation:
  - Vitiligo – consider other autoimmune disease
  - Pityriasis versicolor – loss of pigmentation, like raindrops on the skin; surrounding increase in pigmentation
  - Leprosy – anaesthetic patches, asymmetrical
- Spider naevi – in the distribution of the drainage of the superior vena cava (SVC) – liver disease, pregnancy
- Campbell de Morgan spots – of no significance
- Gynaecomastia – implies an imbalance between oestrogen and testosterone, e.g. hypogonadism, spironolactone
- Neurofibromas – neurofibromatosis (NF) type 1
- Café-au-lait patches – if >5 then associated with NF type 1, as is axillary freckling
- Morphoea:
  - Faintly yellow/ivory thickened skin, either plaques, generalised or linear lesions
  - It does not progress to systemic sclerosis
  - In children and adolescents the 'en coup de sabre' form of linear morphoea may be associated with seizures or headache
- Pattern of hair growth – axillary loss in hypogonadism, or hirsutism in androgenisation, e.g. PCOS
- Striae – livid in active Cushing's, and become silver-like striae gravidarum on removal of excess steroid
- Mycosis fungoides – scaly, erythematous lesions, a cutaneous T-cell lymphoma

LOWER LIMBS

- Moles – the leg is the commonest site for a malignant melanoma in females, the forearm in males; irregular shape and colour, bleeding, itchy, with satellite lesions and regional lymphadenopathy
- Vasculitis – commonly first occurs on the legs
- Erythema nodosum – tender, raised, red lesions; associated fever
- Erythema multiforme – associated mucosal ulceration in the Stevens–Johnson syndrome
- Graves' dermopathy
- Granuloma annulare – diabetes mellitus

- Necrobiosis lipoidica diabeticorum
- Ulcers – venous, arterial, neuropathic or malignant
- Pyoderma gangrenosum – inflammatory bowel disease

FEET

- Keratoderma blenorrhagica – Reiter's syndrome
- Ischaemia
- Neuropathic ulcers – diabetes mellitus

STATION 5

Skin Scenarios

1. SYSTEMIC SCLEROSIS

Points in the examination

Classified as either limited or diffuse, although there is often overlap.

Limited

- Affecting only hands, feet and/or face
- Tight, thick, shiny skin over hands and fingers (swollen) – sclerodactyly
- Facial involvement – beaked nose, microstomia, often with the presence of telangiectasia; look for calcinosis and digital ulcers
- CREST syndrome – (calcinosis, Raynaud's phenomenon, [o]esophageal dysmotility, sclerodactyly and telangiectasia)

Diffuse

- Diffuse skin changes over trunk
- Joint contractures
- Muscle weakness

Either form may also give systemic disease, although it occurs more commonly in the diffuse subtype. Involvement includes respiratory fibrosis, malabsorption, cardiac involvement, and renal disease (hypertension).

Symptoms

- Joints often swollen and painful with limitation of function
- Raynaud's disease
- GI involvement – swallowing difficulties
- Pulmonary involvement
- Renal involvement may result in hypertension

Investigations

- Full blood count
- U+E
- Immunology
- ANA positive in 90%
- Anticentromere and Scl-70 antibodies

- Barium swallow
- ECG, echocardiography
- Chest X-ray, pulmonary function tests, high-resolution CT scan – pulmonary involvement; CT scan is optimal investigation to determine early fibrosis
- Joint radiology – calcinosis or acro-osteolysis

Management

- Raynaud's disease.
  - Avoid sudden changes in temperature.
  - Stop smoking; wear gloves or use hand warmers
  - Calcium antagonists, e.g. nifedipine.
  - $PGEI_3$ production enhancer, e.g. omega-3-marine triglycerides.
  - Infusion of a prostacyclin or perform sympathectomy.
- Proton-pump inhibitors.
- ACE inhibitors substantially improve the outcome in hypertensive crises.
- For systemic involvement, no drug is of proven efficacy, but immunosuppressants are used, e.g. methotrexate.

Points of interest

The 5-year cumulative survival is 35–75%. Adverse factors are increasing age, male sex, extent of skin, heart and renal involvement. Hypertensive renal crises are an important cause of morbidity. There is no cure.

Morphoea is localised scleroderma of the skin, but which does not progress to systemic involvement. Characterised by thickened, waxy plaques most commonly over the trunk or limbs. Children may have linear lesions on the scalp and face.

2. SYSTEMIC LUPUS ERYTHEMATOSUS (SLE)

Points in the examination

Face

- Butterfly rash – and other sun-exposed areas
- Scales/follicular plugging
- Telangiectasia
- Scarring
- Alopecia – 'exclamation mark' hairs
- Vitiligo
- Oral ulceration

Hands

- Vasculitic rash/capillary dilatation in the nail-bed
- Palmar erythema
- Raynaud's phenomenon
- Arthritis – in a rheumatoid pattern but non-erosive
- Jaccoud's arthropathy – non-destructive 'swan necking' of the joints

Other

- Livedo reticularis
- Cushing's syndrome – iatrogenic
- Mononeuritis multiplex
- Peripheral neuropathy
- Pallor, lymphadenopathy, splenomegaly – haemolytic anaemia
- Thrombosis associated with the antiphospholipid syndrome
- Fever
- Haematuria/proteinuria
- Oedema associated with the nephrotic syndrome ± other signs of renal failure

Aetiology

- Autoimmune connective tissue disease of unknown aetiology
- There is a genetic predisposition (associated with HLA DR2, DR3, B8) with environmental triggers
- Drug-induced lupus is a separate entity – procainamide, hydralazine, phenytoin

Symptoms

- Rash
- Arthralgia
- Vasculitic – gangrene and constitutional symptoms of malaise, fever and myalgia
- Bleeding
- Pleuritic pain
- Neuropsychiatric symptoms, including seizures

Investigations

- FBC – anaemia, thrombocytopenia, lymphopenia
- Reticulocytes – autoimmune haemolytic anaemia
- Direct antiglobulin (Coombs') test – positive
- LDH – elevated with haemolysis
- ESR – raised in proportion to disease activity
- CRP – usually normal
- U+E – renal impairment
- C3, C4 – both decreased in relation to disease activity
- ANA – homogenous, sensitive but non-specific
- dsDNA – very specific but less sensitive
- anti-Smith antibody (Ab) – 100% specific but insensitive
- Antihistone Ab – typifies drug-induced lupus
- Anti-Ro and -La – overlap with other connective tissue diseases (NB. Anti-Ro in pregnancy is associated with complete heart block in the baby)
- Antiphospholipid antibodies, false-positive VDRL and the lupus anticoagulant all typify the antiphospholipid syndrome associated with venous thrombosis

Management

- Avoid sunlight – hats, sunscreen and long sleeves.
- Use topical steroids – for rashes.
- Take antimalarials – hydroxychloroquine and chloroquine.
- For arthritis – take NSAIDs or steroids.
- Severe rheumatological or haematological problems require steroids.
- Immunosuppressants – prescribe oral cyclophosphamide, azathioprine.
- Disease activity is monitored by C3/C4 levels, dsDNA titres, ESR and urinalysis.

3. POLYMYOSITIS AND DERMATOMYOSITIS

Dermatomyositis is the same as polymyositis but with skin involvement.

Points in the examination

- Heliotrope rash round the eyes
- Gottren's papules on the metacarpophalangeal joints (can also affect other extensor surfaces)
- Proximal muscle weakness and wasting with muscle tenderness
- Diffuse calcification within the muscles

Aetiology

- 40% of patients have primary disease with unknown aetiology.
- Associated with malignancy in 10–25% of cases, especially lung and ovary.
- Look for clubbing, Horner's syndrome, ascites, lymphadenopathy or hepatomegaly.
- It is associated with other autoimmune diseases in 10% of cases, e.g. rheumatoid arthritis, SLE and may be part of an 'overlap' syndrome. Look for deforming arthropathy or rashes.
- Juvenile forms are associated with contractures and calcification of the muscle. It accounts for 10% of cases and is not associated with cancer.

Symptoms

- Muscle pain and tenderness with progressive weakness
- Dysphagia – pharyngeal muscle weakness
- Symptoms of the cause – haemoptysis, abdominal distension or joint pains

Investigations

- CK, aldolase, LDH
- EMG – spontaneous, small polyphasic potentials
- Muscle biopsy – inflammatory cell infiltrates with muscle necrosis
- CXR
- Tumour markers, e.g. Ca125, CEA

- Autoimmune profile (ANA weakly positive in 60–70%; anti-Jo-1 is specific, dsDNA, ANA, rheumatoid factor (RF) for associated conditions)
- Respiratory function tests are required as the diaphragm is often involved

Treatment

- Mainly supportive.
- Physiotherapy and exercise to maintain mobility.
- Immunosuppressants are of benefit:
  - High-dose steroids
  - Azathioprine, if steroid-unresponsive.
- Overall, there is a 70% 5-year survival.
- 20% of patients recover fully.

Points of interest

Although malignancy is an uncommon association of dermatomyositis, some factors point towards it:
- Male >45 years of age with dermatomyositis
- Absent autoantibodies
- Poor response to treatment.

4. KAPOSI'S SARCOMA (KS)

Points in the examination

- Raised, red/brown, well-demarcated, vascular lesions of varying size are present.
- Treated lesions become browner and flatter.
- KS occasionally causes marked oedema of the limbs, which is difficult to treat.
- Lung lesions can cause crepitations and haemoptysis.
- GI disease can result in abdominal mass and pain.

Sites commonly affected

- Skin
- Feet (soles)
- Mouth
- Stomach
- Lungs

Symptoms

- The lesions can be painful.
- Systemic disease may cause abdominal pain or haemoptysis.

Investigations

- Biopsy and polymerase chain reaction (PCR) for human herpesvirus-8 (HHV-8 – strongly implicated in HIV-related KS)
- CD4 and viral load
- Endoscopy and bronchoscopy only required if symptomatic

Treatment

- Antiretroviral therapy and intralesional chemotherapy for local disease
- Chemotherapy (liposomal anthracyclines or taxanes) for more severe disease
- Radiotherapy often useful for patients with oedema

Points of interest

KS usually occurs in homosexual males practising anal sex and due to transmission of HHV-8. The incidence of KS has dropped since the introduction of HAART. Antiretroviral therapy alone is often an effective treatment.

5. NEUROFIBROMATOSIS

Divided into types 1 and 2.

TYPE 1 (PERIPHERAL FORM; VON RECKLINGHAUSEN'S DISEASE)

Points in the examination

- *Café-au-lait* spots (6 or more, >15 mm in diameter)
- Two or more skin neurofibromas:
    - Subcutaneous, soft, often pedunculated tumours
    - May form plexiform neurofibromas in deeper tissues
- Freckling, especially in groins or axillas
- Lisch nodules – pigmented hamartomas on the iris – require slit lamp for visualisation
- Bone and lung cysts
- Optic gliomas

The diagnosis requires a minimum of two of the above.

Symptoms

- Skin lesions, visual impairment, epilepsy, symptoms of phaeochromocytoma/hypertension

Complications

- Hypertension
    - Phaeochromocytoma (<5% of cases)
    - Renal artery stenosis
    - Coarctation of aorta
- Nerve root compression from neurofibromas
- Epilepsy

Aetiology

- Autosomal dominant condition
- Loss of tumour suppressor gene (*p21ras*) on chromosome 17

Investigations

- Genetic screening
- 24-h urine catecholamines
- MAG-3 scan (renal artery stenosis)
- MRI brain/spine

Management

- Cutaneous surgery for cosmetic or compressive reasons
- Genetic counselling

TYPE 2 (CENTRAL FORM)

Points in the examination

- Bilateral or unilateral acoustic neurofibromas
- Schwannomas of other cranial nerves or peripheral nerves (less commonly)
- Intracranial tumours:
  - Meningiomas (up to 40%)
  - Gliomas – optic gliomas are the commonest intracranial tumour in children
- Skin abnormalities are less common, but *café-au-lait* patches can occur
- Juvenile cataracts

Symptoms

- Progressive hearing loss, tinnitus and vertigo (uni- or bilateral), symptoms of raised intracranial pressure, visual impairment

Aetiology

- Autosomal dominant
- Loss of tumour suppressor gene on chromosome 22

Investigations

- Genetic screening
- MRI cerebellopontine angle for acoustic neuromas
- Auditory testing

Management

- Surgery
- Genetic counselling

6. XANTHOMAS

There are three clinical settings relating to hyperlipidaemia that one may encounter in PACES, depending on the degree of elevated cholesterol or triglyceride concentrations.

EXTENSOR TENDON XANTHOMAS

Points in the examination

- Classically occur on the back of the hands and Achilles' tendon
- Associated xanthelasma (skin lipid deposit around the eyelids) and arcus
- Signs of associated ischaemic heart disease – bradycardia (β-blockade), sternotomy scar

Symptoms

- Ischaemic heart disease

Aetiology

- Raised LDL cholesterol
  - Type IIA familial hypercholesterolaemia – autosomal dominant disease due to a defect in the LDL receptor (chromosome 19); 0.2% of the Caucasian population

Investigations

- Cholesterol (markedly elevated)
- HDL, LDL, triglycerides
- Family history

ERUPTIVE XANTHOMAS

Points in the examination

- Multiple, small, yellow vesicles on extensor surfaces
- Fundi often reveals lipaemia retinalis
- Hepatosplenomegaly due to accumulation of fat-laden macrophages
- Associated with recurrent pancreatitis
- Signs of diabetes (e.g. ocular, vascular and neurological disease)

Symptoms

- Diabetes, pancreatitis and ischaemic heart disease

Aetiology

- Raised triglycerides:
    - Very low-density lipoprotein (VLDL) – familial hypertriglyceridaemia
    - Chylomicrons – lipoprotein lipase deficiency
- Primary – type IV familial hypertriglyceridaemia and lipoprotein lipase deficiency (autosomal recessive diseases)
- Secondary – associated with poorly controlled diabetes mellitus

Investigations

- Triglycerides elevated
- Cholesterol may be normal
- Glucose; Hb A_{1c}
- Appearance of plasma (lipaemic)

PALMAR XANTHOMAS

Points in the examination

- Yellow discoloration of the palms, often raised, which commonly occurs in the digital creases
- Look at knees for tuberoeruptive xanthomas
- Associated xanthelasma
- Signs of associated ischaemic heart disease or secondary causes (hypothyroidism)

Symptoms

- Diabetes, hypothyroidism, renal disease and ischaemic heart disease

Aetiology

- Raised cholesterol and triglycerides
- Primary – remnant particle disease (type III)
- Secondary – diabetes, hypothyroidism, renal disease

Investigations

- Serum electrophoresis (broad J-shaped band; an intermediate-density lipoprotein (IDL) containing equal cholesterol and triglycerides)
- Floating LDL-like band on ultracentrifugation
- Glucose; Hb A_{1c}
- T_4 and TSH

The Locomotor Examination

Examination of the locomotor system comprises of one of the 5 minute clinical stations in PACES. It will usually involve either examination of gait/posture, with ankylosing spondylitis or proximal myopathy being the most common, or require examination of the hands. The four most common hand diagnoses are:

- Arthritides (rheumatoid arthritis, osteoarthritis, psoriatic arthritis, gout)
- Scleroderma or CREST (calcinosis, Raynaud's phenomenon, [o]esophageal involvement, sclerodactyly and telangiectasia) syndrome
- Ulnar or median nerve lesion
- Wasting of the small muscles.

It is important to ensure the patient is comfortable and to rest hands on a pillow. Expose the hands and forearms up to and including the elbows. A large proportion of the patients may have painful and tender joints and it is therefore imperative to ask about this before palpating the joints, which should be done after careful inspection.

INSPECTION

General

- Peripheral accessories, e.g. walking stick
- Peripheral arthropathies, e.g. knees, ankles

Face

- Systemic sclerosis – tight, shiny, stretched skin with beaked nose ± telangiectasia
- Cushingoid appearance – steroid treatment
- Horner's syndrome – T1 lesion

Hands

Approach the examination of the hands themselves in a logical and ordered manner:
- Nails – pitting, onycholysis, clubbing, nail-fold infarcts, Beau's lines
- Skin – tight shiny skin over dorsum of hand or fingers (scleroderma); tissue-paper thin ± purpura (steroid therapy); surgical scars (joint replacement); tar staining
- Muscles:
    - Bilateral wasting of the small muscles with dorsal guttering (rheumatoid arthritis, syringomyelia, motor neurone disease)
    - Unilateral wasting of the small muscles of the hand (C8/T1 root lesion, e.g. cervical rib, Pancoast's tumour)
    - Unilateral wasting involving thenar eminence (median nerve, e.g. carpal tunnel syndrome)
    - Unilateral wasting sparing thenar eminence (ulnar nerve, e.g. elbow trauma)
- Joints (in order to describe the location of the abnormality accurately, candidates should know the names of the bones and joints):
    - Observe the distribution of any abnormalities – symmetrical (e.g. rheumatoid arthritis) or asymmetrical (e.g. seronegative arthritides); proximal or distal joints
    - Specific deformities, e.g. 'swan neck', 'Boutonnière', Z-shaped thumb
    - Subluxation, ulnar deviation
    - Heberden's nodes, gouty tophi,
    - Signs of inflammation – calor, rubor, dolor, tumor and loss of function
        - NB. rubor is replaced with shininess of the skin in those with dark skin
- Elbows for psoriatic plaques or rheumatoid nodules
- Ears for evidence of psoriasis, or gouty tophi in the helix

FUNCTION

- Ask the patient:
    - To make a fist, then a prayer sign
    - To do up a button on the shirt or hold a pen.

PALPATION (WITH CAUTION)

- Palm – Dupuytren's contracture
- Elbow nodules
- Joints – palpate any swelling to determine whether it is soft and boggy (rheumatoid arthritis) or hard and bony (Heberden's nodes or gouty tophi)
- Skin – tightness or calcinosis in finger pulps (scleroderma/CREST)

It is highly likely that by now the abnormality will have become apparent, but if not, you should proceed to perform a neurological assessment, focusing particularly on the median and ulnar nerves.

Locomotor Scenarios

1. RHEUMATOID ARTHRITIS

Points in the examination

- Symmetrical deforming arthropathy affecting the wrist, proximal interphalangeal (IP) and metacarpophalangeal (MCP) joints; sparing of the terminal IP joints.
- Possible 'swan neck' or 'Boutonnière' deformities; subluxation of the wrist and MCP joints.
- Assess function, e.g. writing, undoing buttons.
- Joints may be warm and tender with boggy synovial thickening.
- Z-shaped deformity of the thumb.
- Ulnar deviation at the wrist and MCP joints.
- Wasting of the small muscles of the hand.
- Look for scars of previous operations/joint replacements.
- Look at the feet; consider knee and neck involvement.
- Check for evidence of systemic steroids (Cushing's syndrome).
- Consider extra-articular manifestations:
  - Rheumatoid nodules/olecranon bursitis at elbow
  - Anaemia (6 causes – chronic disease, GI bleeding from NSAIDs, Felty's syndrome, marrow suppression from gold, and folate deficiency from methotrexate and associated pernicious anaemia)
  - Eyes – scleritis/scleromalacia, or keratoconjunctivitis sicca (Sjögren's syndrome)
  - Skin – vasculitis (nail-fold infarcts/purpura/ulcers)
  - Abdomen – splenomegaly (Felty's syndrome)
  - Respiratory – fibrosing alveolitis/pleural effusion
  - Cardiac – pericarditis/effusion
  - Neurological – carpal tunnel syndrome/peripheral neuropathy/mononeuritis multiplex.

Symptoms

- Joints are painful, swollen and warm.
- Typically affects hands and feet, or occasionally a single joint such as the knee.
- Characteristic morning stiffness is present.
- Insidious onset, but may be rapid.
- Function may be severely impaired.
- Patient may be systemically unwell – fever, malaise.
- May have relapsing/remitting nature.

- Palindromic – individual joints affected sequentially.
- Ask about complications such as pulmonary involvement (e.g. dyspnoea), symptoms of atlantoaxial subluxation (e.g. vertebrobasilar ischaemia, limb weakness) and complications of treatment.

Differential diagnosis

Symmetrical polyarthropathy

- Viral – commonly after rubella in young women, 2 weeks after the rash
- Bacterial – e.g. after salmonella enteritis
- Psoriatic arthritis (p. 376)
- Still's disease
- SLE – a non-deforming polyarthropathy (see p. 353)
- Osteoarthritis – completely different pattern of joint involvement

Monoarthritis

- Septic arthritis must be excluded
- Gout/pseudogout

Proximal arthropathy

- Reiter's syndrome – proximal arthritis, commonly knees; urethritis and conjunctivitis ('cannot see, pee or bend the knee')
- Gonococcal arthritis – migratory, asymmetrical; pustular rash near affected joints
- Enteropathic synovitis – in association with ulcerative colitis or Crohn's disease
- Ankylosing spondylitis – back pain and stiffness are characteristic

Investigations

- X-ray of joints involved – periarticular osteoporosis, erosions around affected joint, joint-space narrowing, cysts
- ESR/CRP – evidence of inflammation
- Rheumatoid factor – positive in 80%
- ANA – positive in 30%
- FBC – anaemia of chronic disease, iron deficiency (NSAIDs), neutropenia (Felty's syndrome), associated pernicious anaemia
- CXR – effusion, nodules, fibrosis
- Urinalysis – haematuria, proteinuria

Management

- Diet and lifestyle – light activity and exercise are encouraged.
- NSAIDs – these are the mainstay of initial treatment but give a variable response.
- Disease-modifying antirheumatic drugs – methotrexate or gold – should be used early.
- Immunosuppressants – are also often required in patients poorly responsive to NSAIDs, e.g. sulfasalazine or steroids (monitor for blood dyscrasias and liver function).
- Third-line drugs are hydroxychloroquine, penicillamine, systemic steroids.
- Anti-TNF monoclonal antibody (etanercept or infliximab) result in a significant improvement in severity of arthritis.

2. GOUT

Points in the examination

Arthropathy

- Asymmetrical swelling of the small joints of the hand and feet
- Joint deformity
- Gouty tophi in helix of ear, elbow
- May have olecranon bursitis

Aetiology

- Myeloproliferative or lymphoproliferative disease – e.g. hepatosplenomegaly; lymphadenopathy
- Renal failure – e.g. fistulas, transplant

Symptoms

- The classic presentation is acute pain in a single joint, usually the big toe, often starting at night, which is swollen and exquisitely tender.
- There may be mild systemic disturbance.
- Polyarticular attacks may occur in the minority.
- Attacks are often precipitated by surgery or intercurrent illness.
- Primary gout is due to a genetic disorder of urate metabolism; secondary gout may be precipitated by thiazide diuretics, aspirin, renal impairment, high purine diet or malignancy (high cell turnover).

Differential diagnosis

- Septic arthritis
- Pyrophosphate arthritis ('pseudogout') – usually monoarthritis of major joints
- Rheumatoid arthritis (for chronic gout)

Investigations

- Polarised light microscopy reveals needle-shaped negatively birefringent crystals in the synovial fluid; this is the 'gold standard' diagnostic test
- FBC
- U+E
- Serum uric acid – may be normal during an acute attack
- Urinary urate excretion – differentiates overproducers from under-excretors
- Radiology – characteristic periarticular erosions without surrounding osteoporosis; soft-tissue swelling

Management

- Reduction in weight, alcohol and protein intake (high in purines)

Medical treatment

- Acute attack – give NSAIDs (e.g. indometacin) and colchicine; latter may cause nausea and diarrhoea.
- Prophylaxis – allopurinol lowers serum uric acid levels and is useful in hyperuricaemia; patients will need a prophylactic NSAID at start of therapy.
- Treat secondary causes.

3. PSORIATIC ARTHRITIS

Points in the examination

There are five patterns of disease, of which the classic is:
- Peripheral asymmetrical polyarthritis, affecting the distal interphalangeal joints of the hands and feet:
  - Often associated with 'sausage 'digits – dactylitis
  - Psoriatic nails (onycholysis, pitting, ridging)
  - Skin lesions on extensor surfaces, especially at elbows and knees (absent nodules), behind the ears and scalp.

Other patterns of disease are:

- Arthritis mutilans (telescoping of fingers and toes)
- Symmetrical proximal arthropathy of the hands resembling rheumatoid arthritis but with negative rheumatoid factor
- Sacroiliitis, similar to ankylosing spondylitis
- Inflammatory oligoarthritis – reflecting mainly lower limbs but asymmetrical

Symptoms

- Relating to skin rash of psoriasis
- Of arthropathy

Investigations

- ESR and CRP – guide to disease activity
- Absent rheumatoid factor
- Radiology usually shows asymmetrical small-joint changes with a tendency to ankylosis; often osteolysis, 'pencil-in-cup' deformity

Management

- Activity should be encouraged.

Medical therapy

- Give NSAIDs and analgesia.
- Second-line therapy, e.g. sulfasalazine (nausea, reversible azoospermia, bone marrow suppression); methotrexate (nausea, liver damage, bone marrow suppression); azathioprine (bone marrow suppression), or ciclosporin (impaired renal function).
- Provide skin treatment (e.g. dithranol or coal tar).

Points of interest

- Only 5% of patients with psoriasis develop arthritis.

4. ANKYLOSING SPONDYLITIS

Points in the examination

- Physical signs may be absent when the patient is sitting in a chair
- On standing the signs become evident – the typical 'question mark' posture
  - thoracic kyphosis
  - neck hyperextension – to keep the visual axis horizontal
  - loss of lumbar lordosis.
- Loss of spinal movement
  - Look for loss of lumbar flexion – mark a point between the iliac crests on the lumbar spinous process and a second point 10 cm above this. In a normal individual the two marks will separate to more than 15 cm on full flexion of the spine. In ankylosing spondylitis it is reduced (Schober's test)
  - Restriction of all neck movements.
- Decreased chest expansion with diaphragmatic breathing, leading to a prominent abdomen.
- Central joint involvement – sacroilliitis.
- Peripheral large joint involvement – may be the presenting feature e.g. the knee.

Associated features

- Plantar fasciitis
- Aortic incompetence
- Cardiac conduction defects – look for pacemaker
- Iritis
- Upper lobe pulmonary fibrosis
- Secondary amyloid
- Other spondyloarthropathies
- Psoriasis
- Inflammatory bowel disease
- Beçhet's syndrome

Symptoms

- Back pain and stiffness, worse in the morning, eased by exercise
- Peripheral joint symptoms
- Fatigue
- Dyspnoea

Investigations (initial)

- Spine X-ray – bamboo spine with squaring of the vertebrae
- Sacroiliac joint X-ray – obliteration of the sacroiliac joint
- CRP, ESR – raised
- FBC – anaemia of chronic disease or microcytic associated with NSAID use
- CXR – upper lobe fibrosis
- ECG – conduction defects

Further investigations

- CT chest (high resolution) – fibrosis
- Pulmonary function tests with transfer factor – restrictive defect and reduced gas transfer
- Echocardiography – aortic incompetence, RVH
- U+Es – renal impairment in secondary amyloid

Treatment

- Exercise – maintains function
- NSAIDs
- Spinal surgery – rare.

5. PROXIMAL MYOPATHY

Points in the examination

- Difficulty in rising from a chair or from a squatting position
- Symmetrical wasting and weakness of the proximal muscles
- Reflexes normal – unless the disease is very advanced. This differentiates it from a neuropathy where the reflexes are lost early on
- Faciculations – may be present in advanced disease
- Gait – waddling like that of a duck. The body is tilted backwards with an increase in the lumbar lordosis, the feet are planted widely and the body sways from side to side as each step taken. It is due to difficulty in maintaining pelvic and truncal posture.

Aetiology

- Polymyositis or dermatomyositis – Gottren's pads or heliotrope rash
- Cushing's syndrome (see p. 413)
- Thyrotoxicosis (see p. 405)
- Myasthenia gravis – ocular signs, weak nasal voice, dysphagia, thymoma, fatiguability of power and reflexes
- Lambert Eaton myasthenic syndrome – power and reflexes improve with exercise, associated with underlying small cell carcinoma of the lung
- Dystrophia myotonica (see p. 252–254)
- Muscular dystrophies
- Fascio-scapulo-humeral – wasting of facial and limb girdle musculature, winging of the scapulae
- Limb girdle – spares the face
- Duchenne's – psuedohypertrophy of the calves and buttocks, wasting of the thighs. Gower's sign – climbing up on attempted standing. Heart failure causes death in the 2nd decade
- Alcoholism
- Hypocalcaemia, hypokalaemia
- Ureamia
- Carcinomatosis

Symptoms

- Weakness – difficulty in climbing stairs, rising from a chair, Cossack dancing
- Polymyositis – painful muscles
- Symptoms related to the underlying cause

Investigations

- EMG – there is no denervation; insertional activity and repetitive discharges (polymyositis)
- CK – raised in polymyositis
- Muscle biopsy
- ESR, CRP
- T_4, TSH
- Dexamethasone suppression test – although iatrogenic Cushing's syndrome is most likely
- Anti-acetylcholine (Ach) receptor antibodies
- CXR – thymoma, lung malignancy

Treatment

- Related to cause
- Supportive care

The Eye Examination

It is almost certain that you will be asked to examine the eyes, particularly the fundus, in the PACES examination. Like the other systems, it is considered to be one of the core skills for an MRCP candidate, but one with which many have considerable difficulty. It is essential to practise your fundoscopy technique until it is fluent; by doing so, you will become increasingly confident in your competence to diagnose the relatively few possibilities.

This section should be read in conjunction with that on examination of cranial nerves (p. 204).

OBSERVATION

- Observe the eyes. Look carefully for symmetry involving the eyelids, pupils and general eye movements. In particular, check for signs such as ptosis, lid retraction or irregular pupils. Look around for clues suggesting decreased visual acuity, e.g. white stick, adjacent Braille books; or for evidence of other systemic diseases such as diabetes, e.g. glucose stix, diabetic drinks, foot ulcers or evidence of coexistent dialysis.
- *Visual acuity.* This should be assessed with the patient wearing their normal glasses. Ask the patient if they can see from each eye, and then assess individually by use of a Snellen chart – a pocket one if necessary. Visual acuity is defined as $V = d/D$, where d = distance at which numbers are read and D = that at which they *should* be read.
- *Visual fields.* Visual fields should be assessed by confrontation, with you sitting approximately 1 m from the patient and with your eyes at the same level. When assessing the patient's right eye, ask them to cover up their left eye; after covering your right eye, slowly bring your hand in from the periphery in a plane equal to that between you and the patient. A common error is to bring the hand in too quickly, not allowing the patient time to delineate when they first see it. A red pin should be used for assessing central colour vision that is located around the macula.
- *Eye movements* – see pp. 206–208.
- *Fundoscopy.* This should be performed in a dark room. If not, ask to turn the lights off. A mydriatic will usually have been used. It is essential that you examine the patient's right eye with your right eye

383

and, conversely, their left eye with your left eye. The latter is a routine many candidates have difficulty with, but failure to do this, for whatever reason, is frowned upon. Although the temptation and tendency is to go straight to the retina, you should get into the routine of gradually racking down through the lens strengths: examining first the iris with a positive lens, then gradually examining the anterior chamber, lens and vitreous humour by reducing the strength of the lens. The retina is usually observed with a zero or a slightly negative lens, depending on whether the patient is myopic. The disc and each quadrant of the retina should be identified and studied in turn:

- *Disc* – note its shape, colour (pale in optic atrophy), margins and the presence of papilloedema
- *Retinal blood vessels* – should be examined in each quadrant, noting their diameter (arteries are narrower than veins) and the point at which they cross; look for arterial emboli (arteries become much thinner or thread-like) or venous thrombosis (veins become engorged with surrounding haemorrhages)
- *Retinal quadrants* – each should be examined for the presence of haemorrhages (dot-, blot- or flame-shaped), microaneurysms, pigmentation or exudates – the latter should be identified as hard (white/yellow and shiny with well-defined edges), or soft ('cotton wool spots'); the presence of new vessels should be identified and any previous photocoagulation scars noted
- *Macula* – this should be specifically examined as the surrounding area is a common and important location for diabetic retinopathy
- *Peripheries of the retina* – examine these, looking particularly for evidence of retinitis pigmentosa (q.v.).

STATION 5

Eye Scenarios

385

1. OPTIC ATROPHY

Points in the examination

- Pale disc with well demarcated margins
- Absence of a direct pupillary light reflex but presence of consensual reflex – possible Marcus Gunn pupil in very early disease
- Papilloedema in the other eye – Foster Kennedy syndrome, unilateral frontal lobe tumour causing ipsilateral optic atrophy and contralateral papilloedema

Aetiology

- Multiple sclerosis is the commonest cause – nystagmus, cerebellar signs, pyramidal weakness, sphincter dysfunction
- Optic nerve compression – pituitary tumour or aneurysm
- Glaucoma – cupping of disc margins
- Ischaemic – e.g. central retinal artery occlusion – look for cherry-red macula; temporal arteritis
- Friedreich's ataxia – cerebellar signs, pes cavus
- Paget's disease – large skull, bowing of the long bones
- Vitamin B$_{12}$ deficiency – glossitis, dementia, subacute combined degeneration (SACD)
- Retinitis pigmentosa and choroidoretinitis
- Leber's optic atrophy – especially in males
- Toxins – tobacco, methyl alcohol, lead
- Neurosyphilis
- DIDMOAD syndrome – diabetes insipidus, diabetes mellitus, optic atrophy and deafness

Symptoms

- Visual loss
- Related to the underlying cause

Investigations

- MRI brain and brainstem – MS
- Visual evoked potentials (VEPs)
- Formal visual-field perimetry

- MRI pituitary/hypothalamus
- Alkaline phosphatase
- Glucose
- Serum vitamin B$_{12}$
- Syphilis serology
- Skull X-ray – Paget's
- Intraocular pressures

Management

- Treat underlying cause if possible.

Points of interest

Three types of optic atrophy:
- Primary – without preceding visible change to the disc
- Secondary – to papilloedema from increased intracranial pressure
- Consecutive – following widespread retinal damage, e.g. retinitis pigmentosa/choroidoretinitis.

2. HORNER'S SYNDROME

Points in the examination

- Miosis
- Partial ptosis
- Anhidrosis
- Normal pupillary reflexes
- Enophthalmos
- Blue/grey iris in congenital cases (heterochromia)

Aetiology

The sympathetic innervation of the eye is interrupted. These fibres originate in the midbrain and anterior roots of C8/T1–2, pass into the cervical sympathetic trunk, then to the superior cervical ganglion and enter the skull with the sympathetic chain around the internal carotid artery, before terminating in the eye.

Preganglionic lesion

- Central (unilateral loss of sweating of head and trunk)
- Syringomyelia – bilateral wasting of the small muscles of the hand, dissociated sensory loss, dysarthria, nystagmus, bulbar palsy and reduced reflexes in arms
- MS – optic atrophy, cerebellar and pyramidal signs

Cord lesion

- Diminished sweating of face
- Pancoast's tumour – primary tumour at the lung apex interrupting T1; clubbing, unilateral wasting of the small muscles of the hand, apical lung signs (see p. 24)
- Cervical rib
- Cervical lymphadenopathy – disrupting the preganglionic fibres
- Neck surgery and trauma – scars

Postganglionic lesion

- No unilateral loss of sweating
- Carotid aneurysm
- Retro-orbital tumours

Symptoms

- Migraine which can cause intermittent Horner's syndrome
- History of lung cancer
- Previous cervical sympathectomy

Investigations

- CXR/CT chest
- MRI scan of the suspected area of pathology

Management

- Treat underlying cause, if possible. The patient will usually be asymptomatic from the partial Horner's syndrome.

3. DIABETIC RETINOPATHY

Points in the examination

- Look around for clues immediately – white stick, diabetes book, diabetic drinks, glucometer, diabetic complications – amputation, Charcot's joints, ulcers.
- Distinguish between background, preproliferative or proliferative retinopathy and maculopathy.
- Background retinopathy:
  - Microaneurysms
  - Hard exudates
  - 'Dot and blot' haemorrhages, distributed throughout the retina or around the macula.
- Preproliferative retinopathy – the above, plus:
  - Soft exudates 'cotton wool spots'
  - Flame-shaped haemorrhages
  - Venous beading or loops.
- Proliferative retinopathy – the above, plus:
  - Leashes of new vessels.
- Maculopathy – photocoagulation scars (p. 394).
  - Circinate rings of hard exudates around the macula.
  - Greyish reflection/discoloration at the macula.
- Possible evidence of previous vitreous haemorrhage (loss of red reflex) or previous retinal detachment with consequent widespread visual loss.
- Cataracts – loss of red pupillary reflex.
- Postural blood pressure – orthostatic hypotension can worsen retinopathy.

Symptoms

- Symptoms of diabetic retinopathy are usually not apparent until the macula is involved and often results in irreversible visual loss. Hence the need for regular preventive screening measures.
- Maculopathy should be suspected if there is a marked deterioration in vision with no obvious changes on fundoscopy.
- History of 'floaters' – small or recurrent vitreous haemorrhages.

Investigations

- Glucose, +/– glucose tolerance test,
- HbA1$_c$

Management

- Regular screening should be implemented.
- Photocoagulation is used to treat both macula involvement and proliferative retinopathy.
- Patient should be referred to an ophthalmologist for:
  - Hard exudates near the macula
  - Preproliferative/proliferative retinopathy
  - Maculopathy
  - Unexplained deterioration in visual acuity.

Discussion

The indications for photocoagulation are both maculopathy and preproliferative/proliferative retinopathy. Photocoagulation may either be focal or panretinal; the differential diagnosis is that of choroidoretinitis or retinitis pigmentosa (see p. 393).

4. RETINAL PIGMENTATION

There are four main causes likely to be encountered in PACES: retinitis pigmentosa; choroidoretinitis; photocoagulation scars; and age-related macular degeneration.

RETINITIS PIGMENTOSA

Points in the examination

- Peripheral widespread scattering of black pigment
- Spiculated pattern
- Symmetrical and bilateral

Aetiology

- Idiopathic
- Associated with:
  - Refsum's disease – autosomal recessive; cerebellar syndrome, peripheral neuropathy and cardiomyopathy
  - Laurence–Moon–Biedl syndrome – autosomal recessive; obesity, hypogonadism, dwarfism, mental retardation
  - Usher's syndrome – congenital deafness
  - Kearns–Sayer – progressive external ophthalmoplegia and heart block
  - Bassen–Kornzweig syndrome – abetalipoproteinaemia, fat malabsorption and spinal cerebellar ataxia

Symptoms

- Initially, loss of night vision – rods are affected more than cones as they are peripheral.
- With progressive disease, the pigmentation advances towards the centre of the retina with consequent increasing tunnel vision. The macula is spared until very late. Most patients are registered blind by the age of 40 years.

CHOROIDORETINITIS

Points in the examination

- Asymmetrical, well defined areas of black pigmentation
- Occurs randomly throughout the retina
- Pale areas due to retinal atrophy
- Can be unilateral

Aetiology

- Toxoplasmosis
- Tuberculosis – constitutional symptoms
- Sarcoidosis – lupus pernio, lymphadenopathy, erythema nodosa
- Syphilis
- Behçet's disease – oral and genital ulcers

Symptoms

- Decreased vision

PHOTOCOAGULATION SCARS

Points in the examination

- Localised focal patches of hyper- and hypopigmentation
- Underlying diabetic changes (see p. 391)
- Can be isolated to macula, or more widespread throughout retina
- Usually bilateral

Aetiology

- Diabetes – macular and proliferative retinal involvement

Symptoms

- Patients are often asymptomatic but may have decreased peripheral vision. Photocoagulation of the macula is often associated with visual impairment.

AGE-RELATED MACULAR DEGENERATION

Points in the examination

- Small area of hypo- and hyperpigmentation localised to the macula
- Drusen – pale yellow spots occurring at the macula
- Neovascularisation around the macula

Aetiology

- Uncertain, but possible deposition of lipofuscin within the retinal epithelium. Incidence rises sharply in those over 65 years.

Symptoms

- Deteriorating visual acuity; metamorphopsia, distortion or scotoma. Commonest cause of blindness in the elderly.

5. HYPERTENSIVE RETINOPATHY

Points in the examination

Retinopathy

Grade 1 – narrowing of retinal arteries
Grade 2 – increased light reflex due to atherosclerosis ('silver wiring')
and arteriovenous nipping
Grade 3 – flame haemorrhages and cotton wool exudates; this is
malignant hypertension
Grade 4 – papilloedema

Aetiology (see p. 104)

- Cardiovascular causes – radiofemoral delay, renal bruit
- Endocrine – cushingoid appearance; weakness from hypokalaemia,
  adrenal mass, tachycardia ± postural hypotension
- Renal – palpable polycystic kidneys, AV fistula

Symptoms

- Grades 1 and 2 retinopathy – asymptomatic
- Grades 3 and 4 – headaches and visual reduction

Investigations (see p. 105)

Aetiology

- Explain to the examiners that you would like to measure the patient's
  blood pressure.
- Evidence should be sought for the cause of the hypertension.

Complications

- ECG/CXR and echocardiography all show evidence of LVH.
- U+E – renal impairment occurs as a consequence of hypertension.

Other investigations

- Attend to other risk factors for cardiovascular disease.
- Glucose.
- Fasting lipids.
- Exercise tolerance test (ETT) ± angiography as symptoms direct.

Management

- Gradual reduction in blood pressure; care should be taken in elderly patients with widespread atherosclerosis as too rapid a reduction may lead to cerebral ischaemia.
- Treat underlying cause, if present. Between 85% and 90% of patients have essential hypertension.

The Endocrine Examination

THYROID STATUS

The assessment of the thyroid status of a patient is considered to be a basic clinical skill, and one that should not present too many difficulties provided the following scheme is followed. The most likely scenarios to be encountered in PACES are goitre and euthyroid Graves' disease. For obvious reasons, patients with hyper- or hypothyroidism are unlikely to appear, although it is essential to be competent in demonstrating these.

Observation

General

Look for signs of thyroid dysfunction:
- Hypothyroidism – pale dry skin, 'peaches and cream' complexion, or dry hair
- Loss of the outer third of the eyebrows is an unreliable and non-specific sign
- Hyperthyroidism – anxious, fidgety patient, 'staring' eyes (lid retraction), sweating, exophthalmos
- Graves' disease.

Hands

- Shake their hands – are they warm and sweaty or cool and dry?
- Fine tremor – arms fully extended with a piece of paper resting on outstretched fingers.
- Palpate the pulse – rate, rhythm and volume (e.g. brady/tachycardia; atrial fibrillation).
- Thyroid acropachy – only seen in Graves' disease, but extremely rare.
- Tar staining – Graves' ophthalmopathy is worse in smokers.

Eyes

- Lid retraction, indicated by visible sclera above the superior limbus of the cornea. This results from sympathetic stimulation of the levator palpebrae superioris in thyrotoxicosis of any aetiology.

- Lid lag – ask the patient to follow the slow downward movement of your finger at a distance of about 50 cm; the upper lid lags behind the descending eyeball.
- Exophthalmos – sclera visible below the inferior limbus of the cornea with the patient sitting at the same level as yourself and looking straight ahead. This only occurs in Graves' disease (q.v.). Synonymous with proptosis; can be unilateral, although a retro-orbital tumour should always be considered.
- Other features of Graves' ophthalmopathy are:
  - Periorbital oedema
  - Chemosis
  - Conjunctival injection.
- Ophthalmoplegia:
  - Ask the patient to follow your finger (and to comment on the presence of diplopia) as you test all movements of the eye (see p. 206). Limitation of upward gaze is the most common abnormality in Graves' ophthalmopathy. However, the combination of enlarged ocular muscles ± subsequent fibrosis may lead to complex ophthalmoplegia that is not explained by either single nerve or muscle disease.
- Ptosis – a very rare occurrence in either Graves' disease or hyperthyroidism. Its presence should raise the possibility of coexistent myasthenia gravis.

Goitre

Follow the sequence: observation, palpation, percussion, auscultation.

Observation

- Look for any obvious thyroid swelling – nodular or symmetrical?
- Ask the patient to swallow a sip of water and look for upward movement of the thyroid gland. NB. A thyroglossal cyst will move upwards both on swallowing and protrusion of the tongue, and can be transilluminated.
- Scar – is there a previous hemi/total thyroidectomy scar?

Palpation

- Stand behind the patient and gently palpate the gland, located two finger widths below the thyroid cartilage, with one hand on each side and the neck gently flexed.

- If a goitre is present, comment on:
  - Size
  - Consistency (soft – 'like the lips', firm – 'like the tip of the nose', or hard – 'like the forehead' (Besser))
  - Diffuse or nodular?
  - Lymphadenopathy.

Percussion

- Percuss very gently for retrosternal extension of a goitre.

Auscultation

- Bruit – classically occurs in Graves' thyrotoxicosis.

Neuromuscular manifestations

- Reflexes – these are slow-relaxing in hypothyroidism; brisk in thyrotoxicosis.
- Proximal myopathy – thyrotoxicosis. Ask the patient to stand up from a chair unaided.

Legs

- Look for Graves' dermopathy – three forms:
  - Sheet-like myxoedema – diffuse coarse skin with non-pitting oedema
  - Nodular localised – violaceous infiltrative waxy area on the shin, resembling erythema nodosum
  - Horny – papilliform, irregular, firm red dermopathy on shin/upper foot.

Endocrine Scenarios

1. Graves' disease
2. Hypothyroidism
3. Acromegaly
4. Cushing's syndrome

1. GRAVES' DISEASE

Points in the examination

- Thyroid status – can be thyrotoxic, euthyroid or hypothyroid – as a result of the disease itself or treatment
- Presence of goitre – small to moderate size and diffuse
- Lid retraction, lid lag – thyrotoxicosis
- Exophthalmos ± ophthalmoplegia – specific to Graves' disease
- Dermopathy
- Acropachy
- Features of other autoimmune disease, e.g. vitiligo, diabetes mellitus

Aetiology

- IgG antibodies stimulating the TSH receptor

Differential diagnosis (thyrotoxicosis)

Thyroid

- Graves' disease – commonest cause
- Toxic multinodular goitre
- Single toxic adenoma
- Thyroiditis
- Factitious ingestion of thyroxine
- Amiodarone therapy
- Exogenous iodine (Jod–Basedow phenomenon)

Non-thyroid

- Psychiatric disorders, e.g. anxiety states
- Phaeochromocytoma
- Malignancy
- Alcohol withdrawal
- Excess caffeine intake

Symptoms

- Weight loss
- Anxiety, palpitations
- Fatigue
- Tremor
- Sweating, heat intolerance
- Neck swelling
- Staring, gritty eyes

Complications

- Graves' ophthalmopathy: diplopia, visual impairment (if very severe, due to optic nerve compression)
- Cardiac disease: atrial fibrillation and congestive cardiac failure (especially in elderly patients)
- Long-term risk of osteoporosis in untreated/poorly treated thyrotoxicosis

Investigations

- Thyroid function tests – elevated T_4 and/or T_3 with suppressed TSH (a detectable serum TSH level in thyrotoxicosis suggests the very rare pituitary TSH-secreting tumour or thyroid-hormone resistance syndromes).
- Autoantibody titres – thyroid antimicrosomal and antithyroglobulin antibodies are often present, but not always, in Graves' disease.
- Radioisotope scanning – will distinguish diffuse uptake (Graves' disease) from multinodular or single adenoma. Absent uptake in thyroiditis or thyroxine ingestion.
- Ultrasound – confirms size and consistency of the gland.

Management

- Carbimazole or propylthiouracil are first-line medical treatment (p. 331). Either titrate dose by biochemical response, or use 'block and replace' regime. Warn patients of side-effects (rash – approximately 1 in 200; agranulocytosis – approximately 1 in 2,000. Patients to seek urgent FBC if they develop a sore throat or other infection).
- β-Adrenergic blockers (e.g. propranolol) provide symptomatic relief until euthyroid. Often require large doses.

- I-131 (radioiodine): useful for long-term treatment, although 50% will become hypothyroid. Contraindicated in pregnancy and breast-feeding. May exacerbate ophthalmopathy, especially in smokers.
- Surgery: total or subtotal thyroidectomy depending on local practice.

Points of interest

- Management of hyperthyroidism in pregnancy requires specialist advice. The fetus is at risk of either hyperthyroidism (passage of thyroid-stimulating antibodies across the placenta) or hypothyroidism due to transfer of antithyroid drugs. Monitoring fetal heart rate is the best measure of disease activity.

2. HYPOTHYROIDISM

Points in the examination

- Pale skin ('peaches and cream' complexion)
- Cool, dry hands
- Coarse dry hair
- Hoarse croaky voice
- Puffiness of face particularly around eyes
- Bradycardia
- Slow-relaxing reflexes
- Cerebellar ataxia
- Effusions in body cavities (pleural, cardiac)
- Erythema ab igne
- Psychosis/depression ('myxoedema madness')
- Goitre – small, diffuse, firm (Hashimoto's disease)
- Features of other autoimmune disease (e.g. pernicious anaemia, Addison's disease)
- Loss of outer third of eyebrows is an unreliable and non-specific sign

Symptoms

- Weight gain
- Fatigue
- Cold intolerance
- Neck swelling
- Hoarseness of voice
- Aches and pains
- Dry skin, constipation
- Menorrhagia
- Oedema

Complications

- Carpal tunnel syndrome
- Hyperlipidaemia and ischaemic heart disease

Aetiology

- Autoimmune thyroiditis – Hashimoto's disease is the commonest cause in the UK
- Iatrogenic (previous radioiodine therapy, thyroidectomy or thyroid irradiation)
- Iodine deficiency – commonest worldwide
- Antithyroid drugs
- Amiodarone (but more often causes thyrotoxicosis), iodine excess
- Poor compliance with thyroxine replacement
- Lithium
- Secondary thyroid failure (pituitary or hypothalamic disease)

Differential diagnosis

- Depression
- Weight gain due to overeating

Investigations

- Thyroid function tests: T_4 will be reduced with elevation of TSH (in primary hypothyroidism). TSH will be inappropriately low or reduced in secondary hypothyroidism.
- Look for antithyroid antibodies – Hashimoto's thyroiditis.
- Ultrasound – may reveal goitre.
- 0900-h cortisol estimation (exclude Addison's – administration of thyroxine to patients with glucocorticoid deficiency can precipitate a fatal addisonian crisis).
- Lipids.
- FBC (macrocytosis – pernicious anaemia).

Management

- Thyroxine – cautious replacement in the elderly. Treat coexisting ischaemic heart disease or Addison's disease before giving thyroxine.
- Patient is euthyroid when TSH returns to within normal range.
- Measure thyroid function yearly.

3. ACROMEGALY

Points in the examination

Due to excess growth hormone

- Large hands and feet with soft tissue overgrowth
- Prominent supraorbital ridges
- Macroglossia
- Prognathism
- Interdental separation
- Broad nose and coarse facial features
- Sweaty, greasy thick skin
- Hypertension
- Carpal tunnel syndrome
- Multinodular goitre in 10–20%

Due to pituitary tumour

- Visual field defects (classically bitemporal upper quadrantanopia, hemianopia)
- Optic atrophy
- Ophthalmoplegia (cavernous sinus syndrome)

Due to compression of adjacent normal pituitary

- Hypopituitarism

Complications

- Cardiac disease – hypertension and diabetes mellitus are risk factors for ischaemic heart disease; cardiomyopathy also occurs
- Respiratory disease – upper airway obstruction due to macroglossia; goitre and soft tissue enlargement cause obstructive sleep apnoea
- Colorectal adenomas and cancer
- Glucose intolerance

Aetiology

- 99% of cases are due to a pituitary growth-hormone-secreting adenoma.
- Approximately 5% of patients have multiple endocrine neoplasia type-1 (MEN-1) syndrome.
- Very rarely, ectopic growth-hormone-releasing hormone (GHRH) secreted from a neuroendocrine carcinoid tumour (gut, pancreas, lung).

Symptoms

- General coarsening of facial features
- Enlargement of hands and feet
- Increasing ring and shoe size
- Sweating
- Musculoskeletal abnormalities/osteoarthritis
- Carpal tunnel syndrome
- Local effects of pituitary tumour: headache, visual deterioration
- Symptoms of hypopituitarism – decreased libido, secondary hypothyroidism, amenorrhoea

Investigations

Diagnosis

- Failure of suppression of growth hormone (GH) to undetectable levels following an oral glucose tolerance test. This is the 'gold standard' diagnostic test.
- Elevated serum insulin-like growth factor-1 (IGF-1) level – provides confirmatory evidence.

Pituitary

- Pituitary function – basal and dynamic tests for ACTH, TSH and LH/FSH reserve.
- Measure basal prolactin level.
- Imaging – MRI is the investigation of choice – demonstrates tumour size, local invasion and avoids ionising radiation.
- Plain skull X-ray may show enlargement of pituitary fossa and thickening of skull vault.
- Visual field test – formal Goldman perimetry.

Other investigations

- Fasting glucose
- Lipids
- Bone profile (primary hyperparathyroidism – MEN-1)
- ECG/echocardiogram
- CXR
- Colonoscopy
- Sleep studies
- Nerve conduction studies

Management

- Trans-sphenoidal surgery remains the initial treatment of choice in the majority of patients. Success depends on operator skill and pituitary tumour size.
- Medical:
  - Somatostatin analogues (e.g. octreotide or lanreotide) reduce serum GH in 90% of patients and to a safe GH level in approximately 50% of patients. Side-effects are abdominal discomfort and gallstones (approximately 50% by 5 years)
  - Dopamine agonists (e.g. bromocriptine, cabergoline) are effective in only 10% of patients
  - A newly developed growth-hormone receptor antagonist, 'Pegvisomant' is more efficacious, normalising serum IGF-1 in >90% of patients.
- Irradiation:
  - Pituitary external conventional irradiation is indicated for patients unfit for or not cured by surgery. Results in a 50% decline in GH levels by 2 years but with a continuing exponential decline thereafter. Significant risk of late hypopituitarism
  - Stereotactic focused radiosurgery may offer some advantages.

Points of interest

- The association between acromegaly and colorectal cancer has recently become more apparent. It is an age-dependent complication. In previous studies, the majority of acromegalic patients had died by the age of 60 years from other causes. The relative risk for colorectal cancer is approximately 10-fold above the general population and is related to elevated circulating GH and IGF-1 levels, although the precise mechanisms remain unknown. Acromegalic patients should therefore undergo regular colonoscopic screening.

4. CUSHING'S SYNDROME

Points in the examination

Excess glucocorticoids

- Central obesity
- Thin legs and arms ('lemon on cocktail sticks')
- Moon face with purplish plethora
- Agitation – if severe
- Thin skin
- Purpura and bruises
- Hirsutism
- Pigmentation – particularly if due to ectopic ACTH secretion, or severe Cushing's disease
- Short stature – either from a kyphosis due to osteoporotic collapse, or growth failure if Cushing's occurred in childhood
- Hypertension
- Proximal myopathy
- Injection or lipohypertrophy from insulin
- Infections – e.g. tinea
- Buffalo hump and supraclavicular fat pads are unreliable signs

Features of the cause

- Underlying disease necessitating steroid use, e.g. COAD, renal transplant, eczema (topical steroids are often potent)
- Cushing's disease:
  - Bitemporal hemianopia
  - Hypogonadism in males
- Adrenalectomy scar – rooftop, or bilateral loin incisions (unilateral for single adenoma)

Aetiology

- Iatrogenic – the commonest cause, e.g.:
  - Rheumatoid arthritis
  - Psoriasis – topical steroid cream
  - Asthma – inhaled and oral steroids
  - Post-transplant – renal

- Spontaneous Cushing's syndrome (and approximate % of cases)
  - ACTH-dependent disease (80%):
    - Cushing's disease – two-thirds of ACTH-dependent disease
    - ectopic ACTH
    - unknown source
  - ACTH-independent (20%):
    - adrenal adenoma
    - adrenal carcinoma
- Pseudo-Cushing's syndrome:
  - Alcoholism
  - Depression

Symptoms

- Weight gain, particularly centrally
- Change in appearance
- Growth delay
- Loss of height
- Weakness
- Hirsutism
- Acne
- Bruising and thin skin
- Mood change
- Purple stretch marks
- Nocturia/polyuria
- Decreased libido; impotence in men
- Oligo/amenorrhoea in women
- Infections
- Headaches
- Visual disturbance

Initial investigations

- Screening tests – high sensitivity and low specificity:
  - Overnight dexamethasone suppression test (1 mg at 2200 h); normal is an undetectable cortisol at 0900 h the following day
  - 24-h urinary free cortisol
- Confirmation of Cushing's syndrome – low sensitivity, high specificity:
  - Loss of circadian variation in cortisol – detectable sleeping midnight cortisol level (100% specific for active Cushing's disease)
  - Low-dose dexamethasone suppression test – 0.5 mg taken at 6-hourly intervals for 48 hours; serum cortisol level should be suppressed at 48 hours

- FBC, ESR – mild polycythaemia
- U+E including bicarbonate – hypokalaemic alkalosis, especially in ectopic ACTH syndromes
- Bone profile – raised ALP if recent osteoporotic collapse
- LFTs including γ-GT – steatosis is common
- Fasting plasma glucose and serum lipids
- CXR – cardiomegaly, rib fractures, thoracic vertebral collapse, lung tumour
- Lumbar spine XR/DEXA – osteoporosis
- Plasma alcohol – may help in evaluation of alcoholic pseudo-Cushing's syndrome

Once Cushing's syndrome is diagnosed, further investigation is best performed in a specialist centre.

Further investigations (to establish the aetiology)

- Plasma ACTH – will be undetectable in adrenal causes, adenoma, carcinoma
- To differentiate the causes of ACTH-dependent disease:
  - High-dose dexamethasone suppression test – 2 mg at 6-hourly intervals for 48 hours:
    - in pituitary-dependent disease, serum cortisol level at 48 h suppresses by 50%; in ectopic ACTH it fails to suppress in the majority of cases
    - corticotrophin-releasing hormone (CRH) stimulation test – cortisol and ACTH fail to rise in the majority of ectopic ACTH syndromes
    - inferior petrosal sinus sampling with CRH stimulation – confirms Cushing's disease and can aid in tumour lateralisation
    - whole-body venous sampling catheter to locate the source of ectopic ACTH
- Radiology:
  - MRI of the pituitary and hypothalamus – may demonstrate the adenoma in ~50% patients with Cushing's disease
  - CT abdomen – will demonstrate unilateral adrenal disease; look for atrophy of the contralateral adrenal
    - in ACTH-dependent disease both adrenals are enlarged
  - CT chest – for ectopic ACTH, often from a bronchial carcinoid

Management

It is necessarily dependent on the aetiology.

Iatrogenic Cushing's disease

- Minimise dose of steroid, by whichever route, or consider steroid-sparing agents, e.g. azathioprine in Crohn's disease.
- Treat hyperlipidaemia or diabetes mellitus/impaired glucose tolerance (IGT); treat or prevent osteoporosis – bisphosphonates.

Cushing's disease

- Trans-sphenoidal pituitary surgery (TPS) – is the treatment of choice; results in cure in 50% of cases in expert hands.
- Pituitary irradiation – adjunctive to TPS – has the side-effects of hypopituitarism.
- Medical blockade – adjunctive to above – give metyrapone ± ketoconazole.
- Adrenalectomy – unilateral for adrenal adenoma/carcinoma, bilateral for Cushing's disease. The latter necessitates lifelong glucocorticoid and mineralocorticoid replacement, and may be complicated by Nelson's syndrome.
- Adrenal disease – adrenalectomy.

Abbreviations

5-HIAA	5-hydroxyindoleacetic acid
AA	amyloid A (protein)
AAA	abdominal aortic aneurysm
Ab	antibody
ABG	arterial blood gas
ACE	angiotensin-converting enzyme
ACTH	adrenocorticotrophic hormone
ADL	activities of daily living
AF	atrial fibrillation
AFB	acid-fast bacilli
AFP	α-fetoprotein
AL	amyloid L (protein)
ALL	acute lymphoblastic leukaemia
ALP	alkaline phosphatase
ALS	amyotrophic lateral sclerosis
AML	acute myeloid leukaemia
ANA	antinuclear antibody
ANCA	antineutrophil cytoplasmic antibody
anti-GBM	antiglomerular basement membrane
APTT	activated partial thromboplastin time
AR	aortic regurgitation
AR	autosomal recessive
AS	aortic stenosis
ASD	atrial septal defect
ASO	antistreptolysin O
AST	aspartate aminotransferase
AV	aortic valve
AVM	arteriovenous malformation
BIPAP	bilevel positive airway pressure
b.p.m.	beats per minute
BHL	bilateral hilar lymphadenopathy
C	complement
CABG	coronary artery bypass graft
CAD	chronic airways disease
CAL	chronic airflow limitation
CAPD	continuous ambulatory peritoneal dialysis
CCF	congestive cardiac failure
CCU	coronary-care unit
CEA	carcinoembryonic antigen
CF	cystic fibrosis

CFA	cryptogenic fibrosing alveolitis
CFTR	cystic fibrosis transmembrane conductor regulator
CHB	complete heart block
CK	creatine kinase
CLL	chronic lymphatic leukaemia
CLO	*Campylobacter*
CML	chronic myeloid leukaemia
CNS	central nervous system
COAD	chronic obstructive airways disease
COPD	chronic obstructive pulmonary disease
CPA	cerebellopontine angle
CPAP	continuous positive airway pressure
CPR	cardiopulmonary resuscitation
CREST	calcinosis, Raynaud's phenomenon, [o]esophageal involvement, sclerodactyly and telangiectasia (syndrome)
CRF	chronic renal failure
CRH	corticotrophin-releasing hormone
CRP	C-reactive protein
CSF	cerebrospinal fluid
CT	computed tomography
CXR	chest X-ray
DCC	direct current cardioversion
DCM	dilated cardiomyopathy
DIDMOAD	diabetes insipidus, diabetes mellitus, optic atrophy and deafness (syndrome)
DM	diabetes mellitus
DNAR	do not attempt resuscitation
DOT	directly observed therapy
DPTA	diethylenetriamine pentaacetic acid
dsDNA	double-stranded DNA
DVT	deep vein thrombosis
EBV	Epstein–Barr virus
ECG	electrocardiogram/graphy
EDM	early diastolic murmur
EDTA	ethylenediaminetetraacetic acid
EMG	electromyogram/graphy
ENT	ear, nose and throat
ESM	ejection systolic murmur
ESR	erythrocyte sedimentation rate
ETT	exercise tolerance test
FAP	familial adenomatous polyposis
FBC	full blood count
FEV_1	forced expiratory volume in 1 second
FSH	follicle-stimulating hormone
FVC	forced vital capacity

γ-GT	gamma-glutamyltransferase
GBS	Guillain–Barré syndrome
GFR	glomerular filtration rate
GH	growth hormone
GHRH	growth-hormone-releasing hormone
GI	gastrointestinal
GMC	General Medical Council
GnRH	gonadotrophin-releasing hormone
GTN	glyceryl trinitrate
GU	genitourinary
HAART	highly active antiretroviral therapy
Hb	haemoglobin
HCG	human chorionic gonadotrophic hormone
HCM	hypertrophic cardiomyopathy
HDL	high-density lipoprotein
HLA	human leucocyte antigen
HMSN	hereditary motor sensory neuropathy
HNPCC	hereditory non-polyposis colon cancer
HOCM	hypertrophic obstructive cardiomyopathy
HONK	hyperosmolar non-ketotic state
HPC	history of present complaint
HT	hypertension
HTLV	human T-cell leukaemia virus
IBS	irritable bowel syndrome
ICP	intracranial pressure
IDL	intermediate-density lipoprotein
IGF	insulin-like growth factor
IGT	impaired glucose tolerance
IHD	ischaemic heart disease
INO	internuclear ophthalmoplegia
INR	international normalised ratio
IP	interphalangeal
ITU	intensive therapy unit
IV	intravenous
IVC	inferior vena cava
IVU	intravenous urography
JVP	jugular venous pressure
kPa	kilopascal
KS	Kaposi's sarcoma
l	litre
LA	left atrium
LAD	left axis deviation

LAH	left atrial hypertrophy
LAHB	left anterior hemiblock
LBBB	left bundle-branch block
LDH	lactic dehydrogenase
LDL	low-density lipoprotein
LFT	liver function test
LH	luteinising hormone
LKM1	liver–kidney microsomal (antibody)-1
LMN	lower motor neurone
LMP	last menstrual period
LP	lumbar puncture
LSE	left sternal edge
LV	left ventricle
LVEDP	left ventricular end-diastolic pressure
LVF	left ventricular failure
LVH	left ventricular hypertrophy
MAC	*Mycobacterium avium* complex
MAG3	mercaptoacetyl triglycine
MAOI	monoamine oxidase inhibitor
MC+S	microscopy, culture and sensitivity
MCP	metacarpophalangeal
MCPJ	metacarpophalangeal joint
MEN	multiple endocrine neoplasia
MI	myocardial infarction
MLF	medial longitudinal fascicle
MPTP	1-methyl-4-phenyl-1,2,3,6-tetrahydropyridine
MR	mitral regurgitation
MRI	magnetic resonance imaging
MS	multiple sclerosis
MTS	mental test score
MV	mitral valve
MVP	mitral valve prolapse
NF	neurofibroma
NHS	National Health Service
NICE	National Institute for Clinical Excellence
NIPPV	nasal intermittent positive pressure ventilation
NR	normal range
NSAID	non-steroidal anti-inflammatory drug
NYHA	New York Heart Association
OA	osteoarthritis
p.r.n.	*pro re nata* (as required)
PAN	polyarteritis nodosa
PaO_2	partial arterial pressure of oxygen, i.e. arterial oxygen tension

PAS	periodic acid-Schiff (reagent)
PBC	primary biliary cirrhosis
PCOS	polycystic ovary syndrome
PCP	*Pneumocystis carinii* pneumonia
PCR	polymerase chain reaction
PDA	patent ductus arteriosus
PE	pulmonary embolism
PEEP	positive end-expiratory airways pressure
PEFR	peak expiratory flow rate
PET	positron-emission tomography
PG	prostaglandin
PIPJ	proximal interphalangeal joint
PMH	past medical history
PML	progressive multifocal leucoencephalopathy
PND	paroxysmal nocturnal dyspnoea
PPM	permanent pacemaker
PS	pulmonary stenosis
PSA	prostate-specific antigen
PSM	pansystolic murmur
PT	prothrombin time
PTU	propylthiouracil
PVS	persistent vegetative state
RA	rheumatoid arthritis
RAD	right axis deviation
RBBB	right bundle-branch block
RCA	right coronary artery
RF	rheumatoid factor
RFT	respiratory function test
rhDNAase	recombinant human DNase
RV	right ventricle
RVH	right ventricular hypertrophy
SACD	subacute combined degeneration
SAH	subarachnoid haemorrhage
SAM	systolic anterior motion
SBE	subacute bacterial endocarditis
SCDC	subacute combined degeneration of the cord
SIADH	syndrome of inappropriate antidiuretic hormone (secretion)
SLE	systemic lupus erythematosus
SOD-1	superoxide dismutase-1
SOL	space-occupying lesion
SR	sinus rhythm
SSRI	selective serotonin-reuptake inhibitor
SVC	superior vena cava
TB	tuberculosis

TEN	toxic epidermal necrolysis
TENS	transcutaneous electrical nerve stimulation
TIA	transient ischaemic attack
TIPS	transjugular intrahepatic portosystemic stent
T_LCO	transfer factor for carbon monoxide
TNF	tumour necrosis factor
TPS	trans-sphenoidal pituitary surgery
TR	tricuspid regurgitation
TSH	thyroid-stimulating hormone
TT	thrombin time
TV	tricuspid valve
TVF	tactile vocal fremitus
U+E	urea plus electrolytes
UC	ulcerative colitis
UKPDS	UK Prospective Diabetes Study
UMN	upper motor neurone
URTI	upper respiratory tract infection
UTI	urinary tract infection
V/Q	ventilation–perfusion
VDRL	Venereal Disease Research Laboratories (test for syphilis)
VEP	visual evoked potential
VER	visually evoked response
VLDL	very low-density lipoprotein
VR	vocal resonance
VSD	ventricular septal defect
VT	ventricular tachycardia
WPW	Wolff–Parkinson–White

Biographical Notes

Achilles (early 12th century B.C.), son of Peleus, King of the Myrmidons and the Nereid, Thetis. Brought up by his mother at Phthia, his mother attempted to make him immortal by dipping him in the river Styx, holding him by the ankle. He was the greatest of the Greek heroes in the Battle of Troy; having slain Hector he was killed when an arrow fired by Priam's son, Paris, and guided by Apollo, struck him in the ankle.

Adams, R. (1791–1875), Irish surgeon. Regius Professor of Surgery at University of Dublin and surgeon to the Queen. Famous for his work on gout.

Addison, Thomas (1795–1860), physician at Guy's Hospital, London. Perhaps the greatest of the Guy's triumvirate of Addison–Bright–Hodgkin. After a short note in the *London Medical Gazette* about a new form of anaemia associated with disease of the suprarenal glands (perhaps pernicious anaemia), he followed this up with his monograph *On the Constitutional and Local Effects of Disease of the Suprarenal Capsule*. Initially much discounted in England and Scotland, Trousseau in Paris was quick to recognise adrenal failure and gave it the eponym 'Addison's disease'.

Adie, William John (1886–1935), British physician and neurologist. Mentioned in dispatches in 1916 for saving the lives of a number of soldiers in one of the early gas attacks by improvising a mask of clothing soaked in urine.

Babinski, Joseph Jules François Félix (1857–1932), Head of the Neurological Clinic, Hôpital Pitié, Paris.

Barr, Yvonne, contemporary British virologist, who together with Sir Michael Epstein was the first to isolate herpesvirus from cultured Burkitt's lymphoma cells.

Barré, Jean Alexandre (1880–1967), French neurologist.

Beau, Joseph Honoré Simon (1806–1865), Paris physician. Gave the first description of cardiac insufficiency and asystole, sometimes called Beau's syndrome.

Behçet, Hulusi (1889–1948), Turkish dermatologist.

Bell, Sir Charles (1774–1842), Scottish anatomist, surgeon and physiologist. Founded the Middlesex Hospital and Medical School. Leaving London in 1836 to become Professor of Surgery in Edinburgh, he said, 'London was a good place to live in but not to die in' – also returned to Edinburgh for his love of fly-fishing.

Besser, G. Michael (b. 1936), contemporary physician. Emeritus Professor of Endocrinology, St Bartholomew's Hospital.

Biedl, Arthur (1869–1933), Professor of Physiology, Prague.

Broca, Pierre P. (1824–1880), Professor of Clinical Surgery, Paris.

Budd, George (1808–1882), Professor of Medicine, King's College Hospital, London. His work on the liver started when physician at the Dreadnought Hospital Ship, where he treated innumerable sailors with liver disease on their return from the tropics.

Calmette, Léon Charles Albert (1863–1933), French physician and bacteriologist. Famous for the ground-breaking research that lead to the Bacillus Calmette–Guérin vaccine with Jean-Marie Camille Guérin (q.v.).

Celsus, Aurelius C. (C. A.D. 25), Roman encyclopedist and medical author. He first expounded the cardinal signs of inflammation that bear his name.

Charcot, Jean-Martin (1825–1893), Physician, Hôpital Salpêtrière, Paris. Founder of modern neurology, with incomparable qualities as teacher, writer and organiser that contributed most to his great reputation as a gifted clinician. Lover of animals, his antipathy against Englishmen probably stemmed from his disgust at fox-hunting.

Chiari, Hans (1851–1916), Professor of Pathology, Prague. Made careful use of interesting specimens at postmortem for his own teaching and the museum.

Coombs, Robert Royston Amos (b. 1921), UK immunologist: said "erythrocytes were primarily designed by God as tools for the immunologist and only secondarily as carriers of haemoglobin."

Corrigan, Dominic J. (1802–1880), Irish physician. In 1832, he published *On Permanent Patency of the Mouth of the Aorta, or Inadequacy of the Aortic Valve*, describing the pulse as part of his study of AR. He invented the Corrigan button, a small circular metal plate with a handle, which when heated and touched on the course of the sciatic nerve acted as a counter-irritant for the treatment of sciatica. He became Physician to Queen Victoria in 1847, and was elected President of the Irish College of Physicians in 1859, and remained so until 1863. While President, it became the first College in the British Isles to admit women to the licence examination, thus enabling them to enrol on the medical register, although they could not become Fellows until 1924!

Crohn, Burill Bernard (1884–1956), US gastroenterologist. Persuaded by a colleague to change the name from terminal ileitis to regional ileitis before he first presented the disease that subsequently bore his name.

Cushing, Harvey (1869–1939), US neurosurgeon. Pioneer, who reduced the mortality of neurosurgery for tumours from almost 100% to less than 10%; the mecca of neurosurgery was in his clinics.

de Musset, Alfred (1810–1857), French poet. The sign was first mentioned by his brother Paul in his biography about Alfred. Paul and his mother noticed it while having breakfast with Alfred in 1842. On mentioning it, Alfred put his finger and thumb on his neck and his head stopped bobbing.

Descemet, Jean (1732–1810), Parisian surgeon and anatomist.

Doppler, Christian Johann (1803–1853), Austrian physicist and mathematician.

Down, John Langdon Haydon (1828–1896), English physician. Student of and assistant physician to The London Hospital, also superintendent at Earlswood Asylum where he worked for the hitherto neglected mentally retarded children.

Drager, Glenn Albert (1917–1967), US neurologist.

Dupuytren, Baron Guillaume (1777–1835), French surgeon. 'The beast at the Seine', 'The brigand of the Hôtel-Dieu', 'The miser who would give the king one million francs', 'First among surgeons', 'Last among Men', 'The Napoleon of surgery'.

Duroziez, P. L. (1826–1897), French general practitioner. Noted for his articles on mitral stenosis and other cardiac disorders. President de Societé de Medicine (1882), and Chevalier de la Legion d'honneur (1895).

Eaton, Lealdes McKendree (1905–1958), US neurologist.

Ebstein, Wilhelm (1836–1912), German physician. Made many contributions to studies of metabolic and cardiac diseases.

Eisenmenger, Victor (1864–1932), German physician.

Epstein, Sir Michael Anthony (b. 1921), UK pathologist.

Fallot, E. L. A. (1850–1911), French physician.

Felty, Augustus Roi (1895–1964), US physician.

Fisher, Charles Miller, contemporary Canadian neurologist. Observed that narrowing of the carotid artery caused stroke, and described transient ischaemic attacks from warning showers off clots.

Fleischer, Bruno (1874–1965), German ophthalmologist.

Flint, Austin (1812–1886), American physician. First described the hepatorenal syndrome.

Foville, Achille-Louis-François (1799–1878), French neurologist and psychiatrist.

Friedreich, Nikolaus (1825–1882), German physician.

Froment, Jules (1878–1946), French physician.

Galen (c. A.D. 130–200), physician to three successive Roman emperors.

Gaucher, Phillipe Charles Ernst (1854–1918), Paris physician.

Gottren, Heinrich Adolf (1890–1974), German dermatologist.

Gram, Hans Christian Joachim (1853–1938), Danish pharmacologist, pathologist and bacteriologist.

Graves, Robert James (1797–1853), Irish physician. Besides his disease he also described angioneurotic oedema, scleroderma, erythromyalgia and the pinhole pupil from pontine bleeding. Sometimes sarcastic; in dealing with a colleague's attack on the use of the stethoscope which he and Stokes advocated, he wrote, 'We suspect Dr Clutterbuck's sense of hearing must be injured: for him the "ear trumpet" magnifies but distorts sound, rendering it less distinct than before.' (Henry Clutterbuck (1770–1856))

Gubler, Adolphe-Maire (1821–1897), French physician and pharmacologist. First to distinguish between haemolytic and hepatic icterus.

Guérin, Jean-Marie Camille (1872–1961), French veterinary surgeon. Famous for the ground-breaking research that led to the Bacillus Calmette–Guérin vaccine. He suggested that TB grown on bile would become less virulent, probably first postulated with Kristian Feyer Andvord (1855–1934) when in Paris during 1914.

Guillain, Georges (1876–1961), French neurologist.

Gunn, Robert Marcus (1850–1909), London ophthalmologist.

Hallpike, Charles (1900–1979), English ear, nose and throat surgeon.

Hamman, L. V. (1877–1946), US physician.

Hashimoto, Hakura (1881–1934), Japanese surgeon.

Heberden, William (1710–1801), English physician. His commentary on the *History and Cure of Diseases* was the last important treatise written in Latin in the last 20 years of his life. In the Foreword he reminds us of Plutarch's description of the Vestal Virgins, whose lives were separated into three periods: the first devoted to acquiring knowledge of the duties of her position; the second to exercising these duties; the third to teaching them to others. He felt Plutarch's description may serve as an example for the career of physicians.

Hodgkin, Thomas (1798–1866), Guy's Hospital, London, physician and most prominent British pathologist of his time. Described his disease in 1832. Unpopular with the Board at Guy's because of his liberal and stubborn views, he was denied professional advancement. Despite his reputation in London, he made no success of practice – having sat up all night with a wealthy patient, he was given a blank cheque which he filled in for £10, saying the man did not look like he could afford more; the patient did not consult him again. Many friends would not consult him as he would not accept a fee. Published a paper on AR 20 years before Corrigan; described the biconcavity of the RBC and the first case of appendicitis where perforation was noted to be the cause of death. The obelisk, erected by his friend Sir Moses Montefiore on his now forgotten and overgrown grave in Jaffa, bears the inscription 'Here rests the body of Thomas Hodgkin M.D. of Bedford Square, London. A man distinguished alike for scientific attainments, medical skills and self-sacrificing philanthropy.'

Hoffman, Johann (1857–1919), German neurologist.

Holmes, Sir Gordon Morgan (1876–1965), Irish neurologist.

Horner, Johann Friedrich (1831–1886), Swiss ophthalmologist. Established that red–green colour blindness was sex-linked.

Hunt, James Ramsay (1872–1937), US neurologist.

Hunter, John (1728–1793), Scottish anatomist and surgeon. Perhaps the greatest anatomist of all time, founded experimental pathology and put surgery on a scientific footing that laid the foundations for the 20th century's developments. 'Don't think, try the experiment', sums up his attitude which inspired generations of modern surgeons. His marriage was delayed due to his experiments on venereal disease. He believed two diseases could not exist in the same organ at the same time; thus gonorrhoea and syphilis were thought to be different symptoms of the same disease. He lanced his own glans and prepuce to inoculate himself with some fluid from a lesion found on a prostitute. Unfortunately for Hunter, and medicine for years to come, she had both syphilis and gonorrhoea – which were, and continued to be, thought of as the same disease. There is some doubt as to whether this actually occurred, but the cure is said to have taken 3 years. He paid £500 for the body of an Irish giant, who had wished to be buried at sea, to form part of his massive comparative anatomical collection. Died after an argument with the Board of St George's Hospital, and was buried initially in St Martin's in the Fields. His body was later moved, to be one of only three doctors buried in Westminster Abbey.

Huntington, George Sumner (1850–1916), US general practitioner. He first became fascinated with the disease while making calls with his father in East Hampton on the Long Island coast. Its distribution in the world is among Europeans and their emigrants to the New World and Commonwealth.

Hurler, Gertrude (1889–1965), German paediatrician.

Jaccoud, S. (1830–1913), French physician.

Janeway, Edward (1841–1911), US physician.

Jeghers, Harold Joseph (1904–1990), US physician.

Jendrassik, Ernst (1858–1921), Budapest physician.

Johnson, Frank Chamberliss (1894–1934), US physician.

Kallmann, Franz Josef (1897–1965), German–American psychiatrist and geneticist. One of the first to demonstrate a genetic basis of psychiatric disease. Opposed compulsory sterilisation of psychotic patients in Nazi Germany with great censure – banned from talking at meetings or publishing, he moved to the US. Initially, after the war, his US colleagues refused to accept that genetics had an influence on human behaviour, partly because it was taboo and many feared repetition of one of the doctrines of Nazi Germany.

Kaposi, Moritz Kohn (1837–1902), Austrian dermatologist. Described the sarcoma that bears his name in 1892.

Kartagener, Manes (1897–1975), Swiss physician.

Kayser, Bernhard (1869–1954), German ophthalmologist.

Kennedy, Robert Foster (1884–1952), British–American neurologist, Chevalier de la Légion d'honneur. One of the first to use ECT in the management of psychosis, and was the first to point out that shell shock was hysteria – believing it rose from an insoluble conflict between the soldier's instinct for self-preservation and his herd instinct.

Kerley, P. J. (1900–1979), British neurologist. After graduating he spent a year in Vienna, the then centre of world radiology. Joint author of an authoritative text on radiology.

Kerns, Thomas P., contemporary US ophthalmologist.

Korsakoff, Sergei Sergeyevich (1854–1900), Russian psychiatrist.

Kussmaul, Adolf (1822–1902), German physician.

Kveim, Morten Angsar (1892–1966), Norwegian pathologist.

Lambert, Edward Howard, contemporary US neurophysiologist.

Lancefield, Rebecca Craighill (1895–1981), American bacteriologist. Professor of Microbiology at the Rockefeller Institute. Spent most of her life studying various aspects of streptococci.

Langerhans, Paul (1847–1888), German pathological anatomist. Pioneered microscopic anatomy. Best known for his work on the pancreas, but also made discoveries that led to the demonstration of the reticuloendothelial system.

Lasègue, Charles E. (1816–1883), Professor of Medicine, Paris.

Laurence, John (1830–1874), London ophthalmologist.

Leber, Theodor (1840–1917), German ophthalmologist.

Lévy, Gabrielle (1886–1935), French neurologist.

Lewy, Friedrich H. (1885–1950), German neurologist, Professor Extraordinary in Berlin. Fled Nazi Germany to America.

Lhermitte, J. L. (1877–1959), French neurologist and neuropsychiatrist.

Louis, Antoine (1723–1792), French surgeon, physiologist and historian. Was at the forefront of the struggle to free Parisian surgeons from the grasp of the domineering physicians; submitted his M.D. dissertation in Latin, demonstrating that surgeons were as liberally educated as their physician peers. Shortly before his death he began construction of an executing machine with Joseph Ignace Guillotine (1738–1814) that bears his co-inventor's name.

Mallory, Frank (Mallory body) (1826–1941) American pathologist.

Mantoux, Charles (1877–1947), French physician. Championed the use of intradermal tuberculin testing, completely superseding subcutaneous tests. The Mantoux test was, however, invented by Felix Mendel (1862–1925), a German physician.

Marfan, E. J. A. (1858–1942), pioneer of clinical paediatrics in France.

Marie, Pierre (1853–1940), Parisian neurologist and pupil of Charcot.

McArdle, Brian, contemporary British paediatrician.

Millard, Auguste Louis Jules (1830–1915), French physician.

Moon, Robert Charles (1844–1914), US ophthalmologist.

Müller, H. (1820–1864), German anatomist.

Nelson, Don H. (1906–1964), US endocrinologist.

Noonan, Jacqueline Anne (b. 1928), contemporary US paediatric cardiologist.

Olszewski, J. (1913–1966), Canadian neurologist. In 1964, together with Steele (q.v.) and Richardson (q.v.) described the syndrome that bears their names.

Osler, Sir William Bt (1849–1919), Canadian physician and Regius Chair of Medicine at the University of Oxford. Upon leaving Johns Hopkins in 1905, he gave a farewell lecture in which he referred to the 'relative uselessness of men over forty years of age'. Founder of clinical bedside medicine – 'To study medicine without books is like going to sea on uncharted waters; to study medicine without patients is like not going to sea at all.'

Paget, Sir James Bt (1814–1899), surgeon at St Bartholomew's Hospital, London. Outstanding surgeon of his day. Appointed serjeant-surgeon to the Queen in 1877.

Pancoast, Henry K. (1875–1939), US radiologist. Professor of Roentgenology, Philadelphia.

Parinaud, Henri (1844–1905), Father of French ophthalmology.

Parkinson, James (1755–1824), general practitioner, Hoxton Square, London. Published the famous essay on the shaking palsy, he called it 'paralysis agitans', in 1817. Charcot (q.v.) added one more feature, 'rigidity', and attached the eponym 'Parkinson's disease'. Little recognised in England at the time as he was an outspoken critic of the Pitt Government and a member of the secret 'London Corresponding Society', which in 1794 was charged with complicity in an alleged plot to kill King George III – the so-called 'popgun plot', as it was alleged the plan was to fire a poison dart from a popgun at the King in a theatre.

Peutz, Johannes Laurentius Augustinus (1886–1957), Dutch physician.

Phalen, George S. (1911–1998), US orthopaedic surgeon.

Pott, Percival (1714–1788), surgeon, St Bartholomew's Hospital, London. Described painful deformity of the spine with paraplegia, which he considered to be due to tuberculosis.

Quincke, H. I. (1842–1922), German physician. Student of Virchow. Later Professor of Medicine at Kiel until his retirement in 1908. His most notable contribution was the introduction of lumbar puncture as a therapeutic and diagnostic technique. He diagnosed TB meningitis by demonstrating tubercle bacilli in the CSF. When the technique was first reported, in 1891, it attracted little interest, but over the years he saw it become the premier diagnostic technique in neurology.

Raynaud, Maurice (1834–1881), French physician.

Reed, Dorothy (1874–1964), US pathologist, Johns Hopkins Hospital. The first to clearly separate tuberculosis from Hodgkin's disease – maintained that to be Hodgkin's disease 'her' cells had to be present.

Refsum, Sigvald (b. 1907), Norwegian neurologist.

Reiter, H. C. (1881–1969), German physician. Whilst with the 1st Hungarian Army on the Western Front in 1916, he described a young lieutenant with diarrhoea and associated urethritis, conjunctivitis and arthritis. This condition had in fact been reported by Sir Benjamin Brodie (1783–1862) in his 1818 textbook *Diseases of the Bones and Joints*.

Rendu, Henri Jules Lois Marie (1844–1902), French physician and botanist. Compiled one of the finest collections of plants in France.

Rich, A. R. (1893–1968), US pathologist.

Richardson, J. C. (b. 1909), Canadian neurologist. In 1964, together with Steele (q.v.) and Olszewski (q.v.), described the syndrome that bears their names.

Rinne, Friedrich Heinrich Adolf (1819–1868), German ear, nose and throat surgeon.

Robertson, Douglas Argyll (1837–1909), Scottish ophthalmic surgeon.

Roger, H. L. (1809–1891), French paediatrician.

Romberg, Mortz Heinrich (1795–1873), German neurologist and Professor of Medicine in Berlin. Described what is now known as Romberg's sign in tabes dorsalis in his text of 1840–1846, the fist systematic book on neurology.

Roussy, Gustave (1874–1948), French neuropathologist. First to show that damage to the hypothalamus could cause polyuria, obesity, transient glycosuria and even gonadal atrophy.

Sayre, George P., contemporary US ophthalmologist.

Sézary, A. (1880–1956), French dermatologist.

Shy, George Milton (1919–1967), US neurologist.

Sjögren, Henrik Samuel Conrad (1899–1986), Swedish ophthalmologist.

Snellen, Hermann (1834–1908), Dutch ophthalmologist.

Starr, A. (b. 1926), contemporary US physician.

Steele, J. C. Canadian neurologist. In 1964, together with Richardson (q.v.) and Olszewski (q.v.), described the syndrome that bears their names.

Steell, Graham (1851–1942), Scottish physician.

Sternberg, Carl (1872–1935), Austrian pathologist.

Stevens, Albert Mason (1884–1945), New York paediatrician.

Still, Sir George Frederick (1868–1941), first Professor of Paediatrics in England. Along with Maurice Raynaud and Howard Henry Tooth shared the distinction of having an eponym named after an M.D. thesis. His sister-in-law said, 'He loved children, but with the exception of his own mother and the Queen I have never heard him utter a favourable word on mothers in general'.

Stokes, W. (1804–1878), Irish physician. President of the Irish Royal College of Physicians. He is said to have commented, 'My father left me but one legacy, the blessed gift of rising early'.

Sturge, William Allen (1850–1919), British physician and archaeologist.

Tinel, Jules (1879–1952), French neurologist. Took an active part in the resistance against German occupation during the Second World War. He and his family were imprisoned, his son dying in the death camp of Dora.

Todd, Robert (1809–1860), Irish physician and FRS. Founder of King's College Hospital.

Tooth, Howard Henry (1856–1926), London physician.

Traube, L. (1818–1876), German physician. Studied in Breslau with Purkinje and in Berlin under Müller and Schönlein. Introduced the routine use of the thermometer in the examination of his patients in 1850.

Troisier, Charles Émile (1844–1919), French pathologist.

Turner, Henry Hubert (1892–1970), US endocrinologist. One of the founders of modern endocrinology.

Valsalva, Antonio M. (1666–1723), Italian anatomist. Professor of Anatomy at Bologna. Student of Malpighi. Noted that motor paralysis is on the opposite side to the cerebral lesion both in stroke and in cases of cranial injury – a fact confirmed by his greatest pupil, Morgagni, in numerous autopsies.

Virchow, Rudolf Ludwig Karl (1821–1902), German pathologist and statesman. Father of modern pathology, dispelled the last vestiges of humoral theory in medicine and presided over Germany's ascendancy in world medicine after 1840. In 1845, published his classic paper on thrombosis and haemostasis as delineated in his triad, describing one of the first two recorded cases of leukaemia.

von Recklinghausen, Friedrich Daniel (1833–1910), German pathologist. Opposed Koch's view that tuberculosis was due to tubercle bacilli found in the granulomas, saying it was like claiming that the pyramids of horse manure in the Strasbourg streets were due to the sparrows perched on top of them.

Waller, Augustus Volney (1816–1870), English neurophysiologist.

Weber, Frederick Parkes (1863–1962), English physician. Keen alpinist and collector of vases and coins.

Weber, Sir Herman David (1823–1918), German physician practising in London. Father of Frederick Parkes Weber.

Wegener, Friedrich (1907–1990), German pathologist.

Wenkebach, K. F. (1864–1940), German physician. One of the first to recognise the benefits of the vegetable alkaloid quinine on arrhythmias, particularly auricular fibrillation of recent onset.

Wernicke, Karl (1848–1905), Professor of Neurology, Breslau.

Whipple, George Hoyt (1878–1976), US pathologist.

White, Paul Dudley, US cardiologist. In 1955 he attended President Eisenhower during his myocardial infarction, and it is said that only he and the President were convinced that the President would survive.

Williams, J. C. P., contemporary New Zealand physician.

Wilson, Samuel Alexander (1877–1937), neurologist, Queen's Square London. Offered five points of advice based on his experience: (1) Never show surprise; (2) Never say the same thing twice to a patient; (3) Never believe what the patient says the doctor said; (4) Be decisive in your indecision; (5) Never take a meal with your patient.

Wolff, Louis (1898–1972), US physician.

Index

Barnet
Programme